This book is dedicated to late Dr. Kazuhiko Ohashi, for his great achievements Intraductal Papillary Mucinous Neoplasm (IPMN).

Edited by
Makoto Seki, M. D.:
Department of Surgery, Mitaka Center Hospital
Former: Department of Hepato-Biliary-Pancreatic Surgery, The Cancer Institute Hospital of JFCR

Akio Yanagisawa, M. D, Ph. D.:
Designated Professor; Department of Pathology, Graduate School of Medicine, Kyoto Prefectural University of Medicine
Department of Pathology, Kyoto First Red Cross Hospital
Former: Division of Pathology, The Cancer Institute of JFCR

Yo Kato, M. D, Ph. D.:
Professor; Department of Pathology, Dokkyo Medical University Nikko Medical Center
Former: Division of Pathology, The Cancer Institute of JFCR

Kunio Takagi. M. D:
Hayashi Surgical Hospital
Former: Department of Surgery, The Cancer Institute Hospital of JFCR

Published on July 15, 2016 by
IGAKU TOSHO SHUPPAN, Co. Ltd.
2-29-8 Hongo, Bunkyo-ku, Tokyo 113-0033

ISBN978-4-86517-162-4
C3047 ¥5000E

Copyright © 2016 IGAKU TOSHO SHUPPAN, Co. Ltd., Tokyo

No part of this book may be reproduced or utilized in any form or by any means, electronic or mechanical, including photocopying and recording, or by any information storage or retrieval system, without permission in writing from the publisher.

Printed in Japan

Recommendation

Advisor to the Japanese Foundation for Cancer Research

Haruo Sugano

The prognosis of pancreatic cancer is still extremely poor at present. The prognosis was even worse previously, and pancreatic cancer was referred to as being "particularly intractable among intractable cancers."

Even in those days, some members of the Cancer Institute took up the brave challenge of fighting pancreatic cancer ; they were members of the Pancreas Study Group, including Kazuhiko Ohashi (Dept. of Internal Medicine), Kunio Takagi (Dept. of Surgery) and Yo Kato (Dept. of Pathology) and also some members from the Dept. of Radiology. They discussed and reviewed each case with one another. The group meetings were conducted in a very conducive atmosphere for free and active discussions, beyond the border of specialties.

Through continued learning about pancreatic cancer, this group was responsible for several important advances and discoveries. One was full-section round slicing of the pancreas, and another was the discovery of mucus-producing pancreatic tumors. In 1982, Kazuhiko Ohashi et al. reported 4 cases of mucus-producing pancreatic cancer, characterized by mucus production and a unique morphology. Since then, the group has repeatedly published cases of this tumor, reported mucus-producing pancreatic tumors include adenomas and adenocarcinomas, follow the adenoma-adenocarcinoma sequence, and show K-ras mutation. Thus, this tumor began to attract close attention of the medical fraternity as a clinicopathologically independent disease entity.

It is regrettable that during the process of global acceptance of this tumor, IPMN (intraductal papillary mucinous neoplasm) was adopted as its name. But, this does not lower the value of the contribution of Ohashi and other members of the Pancreas Cancer Study Group at the Japanese Foundation for Cancer Research.

Now, publication of an atlas of IPMN is planned, after being edited by 4 researchers of pancreatic cancer (Makoto Seki, Akio Yanagisawa, Yo Kato and Kunio Takagi), who have been involved for many years in research on this disease at our foundation. I am much pleased with this publication.

This atlas is large-sized and splendid, primarily consisting of illustrations. In the Introduction section, the birth of mucus-producing pancreatic cancer and its clinical course are described briefly, followed by a schematic representation of the clinicopathological findings and case groups in parallel, creating quite a striking impression for the readers. In the Case Presentation section, ten carefully selected cases are presented, ranging from typical cases of IMPN to cases of various forms of pancreas cancer which can be viewed as deformed or modified IMPN, arranged in such a way as to facilitate a concrete understanding about the various forms of pancreatic cancer (focusing on IPMN) and the progression of pancreatic cancer. Each case is explained by beautiful graphic representations of the diagnostic imaging, operative and histopathological findings, with comments on the clinical and pathological features provided at the end of each presentation.

This atlas has been prepared based on the principle of "readily understandable by seeing". That is to say, the atlas is designed in a practical manner, with emphasis on the subject at hand, i. e., illustrations. In other words, this atlas is designed so as to let the illustrations speak for themselves. In other words, it can also be easily understood by beginners. At the same time, its contents invite experienced readers into thinking deeper and gain further insight. It is an atlas of such deep taste. It is wonderful.

I recommend this book, and sincerely hope that it will be read and loved by many people.

In the end, I would like to express my respect and gratitude to Mr. Fumiharu Suzuki and Mr. Tomoyuki Kozono of Igakutosho-Shuppan Ltd., for publishing such a precious and splendid book.

I would also like to take this opportunity to talk about Dr. Kazuhiko Ohashi here. We cannot find his name in the list of editors of this book, and unfortunately, he is no more with us. On the occasion of the publication of this book, I would like to propose that this type of pancreatic tumor be called "Ohashi Tumor" in memory of Dr. Ohashi, who was the first to propose this disease entity. I would appreciate your support for this proposal.

Recommendation

Honorary President, Aichi Cancer Center

Yuji Nimura

I offer my congratulations to the authors on the publication of this IPMN Atlas, which presents the history of diagnosis and treatment of mucus-producing pancreatic cancer at the Cancer Institute located at Otsuka.

Around the year 1972-73, when I had training at the Dept. of Surgery, Cancer Institute Hospital, resectable pancreatic cancer had just begun to attract attention. In those days, Dr. Kunio Takagi was actively engaged in the diagnosis of pancreatic cancer by ERCP. Later, Dr. Kazuhiko Ohashi (my classmate at Nagoya University) returned from Sweden and joined the Dept. of Internal Medicine, Cancer Institute Hospital. I think the pair of Takagi and Ohashi accelerated the research on the diagnosis and treatment of pancreatic cancer by eliminating the barrier between the department of internal medicine and the department of surgery in respect of this disease entity.

Even after returning to Nagoya University, I always visited the Cancer Institute during my trips to Tokyo for attending the congresses or research meetings. I made it a rule to join Dr. Tamaki Kajitani, my mentor, on his rounds in the surgical ward, and to visit the offices of Dr. Takagi and Dr. Ohashi to hear the latest updates about pancreatic cancer. Once Dr. Ohashi told me : "Hi, Nimura, I have discovered a strange type of pancreatic cancer." He was still very excited at that time. The tumor he found was later named "mucus-producing pancreatic cancer." Dr. Takagi subsequently published his ERCP Classification, in which mucus-producing pancreatic cancer was categorized as type Ⅲ. Every time I visited the Cancer Institute, I heard Dr. Takagi saying : "I found another case of type III." He would discuss the diagnostic and pathological findings of newly detected cases. Another time, Dr. Takagi showed me an endoscopic picture in his office, saying : "Do you know what this is?" It was a beautiful-color photo showing a papillary growth tumor within the duct. To me, it would be impossible to take such a clear picture by introducing an endoscope so close to the tumor within the fine ductal organ. I imagined it should be a tumor within the pancreatic duct. However, I could not answer a word to him because I thought it impossible to take such a fine picture with a mother-baby fiberoptic-OK endoscope. So, I said : "I can't get it." Dr. Takagi then said : "This is mucus-producing pancreatic cancer." Hearing that, I said, "But, it is impossible to take such a fine picture with a mother-baby fiber scope, isn't it?" Dr. Takagi answered : "This is an electronic endoscopic picture!." "But, there is still no electronic scope that can be used within the pancreatic duct, is there?" To this question of mine, Dr. Takagi revealed the trick, saying : "I observed the lumen of the pancreatic duct of a resected specimen with an electronic scope!" The pictures reminding me of these past episodes are presented in this publication. Such episodes allowed me to take a peek into Dr. Takagi's past research stance, that led to the development of a new diagnostic technology using resected specimens and discovery of new disease entities. When I reviewed my own cases at Nagoya, there was a case of pancreatic head cancer with an enlarged orifice of the papilla of vater many years ago. I remember that on the day before surgery for this case, I performed endoscopy again as it was an unusual case. At that time, I closely observed the orifice of the papilla and looked the deeper part of the main pancreatic duct. When reviewing the history of the research at the Cancer Institute, I would like to note that what is important is whether or not we can imagine a new disease entity when facing an unusual case like this one. I express my respect to the keen eye of Dr. Ohashi who proposed a new disease entity from the intuitive feeling "unusual" and "strange." I reconfirmed that new discoveries may not only be accidental, but also often depend on continuous routine efforts, as commonly seen from the past reports.

If we review the history of pancreatic tumor research from "mucus-producing pancreatic cancer" to "IPMN," we can recognize that various pancreatologists, ranging from clinical specialists to basic scientists, are involved in this research. This atlas makes it clear that this research took its origin in the Cancer Institute at Otsuka, filled with sweat and tears during joint research beyond the barriers of specialties (gastroenterology, surgery, radiology and pathology). There is also the splendid history of identifying the disease entity of "early gastric cancer" from superficial cancer at the Cancer Institute, Otsuka. The research method employed for the proposal of these disease entities at that time was also similar to that used in the discovery of mucus-producing pancreatic cancer.

I pray for the repose of the soul of my good friend Kazuhiko Ohashi and hope that this atlas contributes toward the creation of new disease entities from now on.

Foreword

The successful use of endoscopic retrograde cholangiopancreatography (ERCP), introduced in 1969[1], triggered challenges in the diagnosis of pancreatic cancer, the most difficult among all pancreatic diseases. Based on the efforts made since 1978 for early diagnosis of pancreatic cancer[2] and mucus-producing pancreatic cancer was reported in 1982 as a new entity, and was a report of immeasurable value.

Four cases of this tumor (mucus-producing pancreatic cancer) were reported at the 33rd Kanto Bloc Meeting of the Japan Gastroenterological Endoscopy Society. In the selection of "Excellent Presentation," this report was unfortunately ranked only second, with the presentation of research on malignant gastric lymphoma taking away the award. While this award-winning research did not subsequently cast a significant influence on the research activities within this professional society, the research ranked in the second place attracted close attention as research on a new disease entity among the post-war studies of pancreatic diseases. The name of this disease subsequently spread rapidly across the country like wildfire.

Because this disease was initially reported most often from the Cancer Institute Hospital, it was at first called "Cancer Institute disease", just like in the days when depressed early colorectal cancer (type IIc) was initially called "Akita disease" because it was most often reported from Japanese Red Cross Akita Hospital.

Following introduction of this new disease entity, I think that there was greatest confusion in the field of pathology among the three fields (diagnosis, treatment and pathology), because while pancreatic cancer is often unresectable, surgeons tend to avoid resection in cases with benign pancreatic diseases such as pancreatitis for fear of postoperative complications. Under such a trend of shortage of specimens, there was little opportunity for pathologists to perform microscopy of freshly resected specimens. Therefore, freshly resected specimens of mucus-producing pancreatic cancer (more amenable to resection than other types of pancreatic cancer) and also of freshly resected specimens in cases with difficulty in distinguishing between benign and malignant tumors began to be sent successively to the department of pathology. This probably led to a lot of confusion at the pathology department.

Subsequently, various discussions and debates were held about this new pathological diagnosis. Twenty years after the first report of mucus-producing pancreatic cancer, this type of pancreatic cancer was adopted as an "intraductal tumor" in the histological classification of pancreatic tumors in the General Rules for Surgical and Pathological Studies on Pancreatic Cancer (5th edition, 2002)[3], as shown below.

3. Intraductal papillary-mucinous neoplasms (IPMNs)
    a) Intraductal papillary-mucinous adenoma (IPMA)
    b) Iintraductal papillary-mucinous carcinoma (IPMC)

This disease entity was analyzed in detail based on the clinical and pathological findings from 80 cases encountered at the Cancer Institute Hospital during the 26-year period from 1979 to 2004. This atlas presents the results of detailed evaluations of ten of these 80 cases.

Case evaluation meetings focusing on pancreatic tumorous lesions and involving clinicians and pathologists have been held at the Cancer Institute Hall since 1990 (April 1990 to December 2005, until the 110th meeting). On the basis of cancer mapping using full-section specimens and the findings from full-section histological specimens, including of the ten cases mentioned above included in the atlas, the preoperative diagnostic imaging (ERCP, US, CT, etc.) findings were compared with the histological findings presented on video images.

As for myself, I have been engaged in the research on mucus-producing pancreatic cancer since it was first reported, and it is an unexpected pleasure that the outcomes of subsequent research on the diagnosis, treatment and pathological diagnosis of this new entity has been summarized and published in this book. I sincerely hope that this book will facilitate the diagnosis, treatment and pathological understanding of intraductal papillary mucinous neoplasms of the pancreas (IPMNs) from now on.

Hayashi Surgical Hospital
Kunio Takagi

References

1) Takagi K, Ikeda S, Nakagawa Y, et al : Retrograde pancreatography and cholangiography by fiber duodenoscope. Gastroenterology **59** : 445-452, 1970.
2) Ohashi K, Murakami Y, Maruyama M, et al : Four cases of mucus-producing pancreatic cancer—Focusing on the specific findings from the duodenal papilla. Progress of Digestive Endoscopy **20** : 348-351, 1982.
3) Japan Pancreas Society : General Rules for Surgical and Pathological Studies on Pancreatic Cancer, 5th edition, Kanehara Shuppan, Tokyo, 2002.

Upon publication of this book

Department of Pathology, Graduate School of Medicine, Kyoto Prefectural University of Medicine

Akio Yanagisawa

Clinical and non-clinical research on IPMN is still ongoing, even 30 years after mucus-producing pancreatic cancer was first reported by Ohashi and Takagi et al. in 1982. The information on IPMN contained in this book is the outcome of the long-term accumulation of data on IPMN at the Cancer Institute. The cases covered by this book range from early cases managed by late Dr. Kazuhiko Ohashi as an active internist to the latest case managed by Dr. Seki alone who is one of the editorial staff for this book.

I began to become involved in the pathological diagnosis of pancreatic diseases at the Cancer Institute in 1980. In those days, the pancreas removed from IPMN patients was usually cut by the surgeon along the main pancreatic duct to enable macroscopic observation of lesions within the main pancreatic duct during surgery. For this reason, the main pancreatic duct had already been cut open by the time it was processed by the pathologist into formalin-fixed specimens.

In each of the cases of mucus-producing pancreatic cancer reported in 1982 by Ohashi and Takagi et al., the main pancreatic duct was cut open and photographs of the pancreatic lesions showing papillary growth were presented. For the cases adopted in this IPMN atlas, the main pancreatic duct had not yet been cut by the surgeons, and the pancreatic specimens prepared along the plane rectangular to the main pancreatic duct are shown. At present, pancreatic specimens are usually prepared without cutting the main pancreatic duct, as described in General Rules for Surgical and Pathological Studies on Pancreatic Cancer. In those days, however, the main pancreatic duct was usually opened to enable observation of its lumen soon after resection under the initiative of the surgeons. How did preparation of pancreatic specimens without the main pancreatic duct having been cut become a norm thereafter? It was a result of postoperative conferences beginning to be held among surgeons, internists and pathologists. In those days, checking of the pancreatic duct direction/arrangement by endoscopic retrograde pancreatography (ERP) played an important role in diagnostic imaging of the pancreas. During these aforementioned conferences, it was clarified by the pathologists that pancreatic specimens with the main pancreatic duct already cut made it difficult to compare the pancreatic duct arrangement in relation to the histological findings, therefore, formalin-fixed pancreas specimens without the main pancreatic duct having been cut began to be received from the surgeons. Then, how was the removed pancreas handled in those days? Soon after the start of the conferences, the internist (late Dr. Ohashi) was invited to the operating room soon after resection of the pancreas, and he carried the resected specimen into the X-ray room for postoperative pancreatography by infusing contrast material into the pancreatic duct. The postoperative conferences with pathologists were held twice, i. e., once to discuss the macroscopic findings of the resected specimen and another time to discuss the findings from histological examination of the HE-stained specimens. During these discussions with the clinicians about the preoperative images, postoperative images and histological findings, it was found that self-lysis of tissue was more marked in cases with clearer images on postoperative pancreatography, with the intraductal papillary structure in IPMN cases becoming almost invisible during histological examination. This was a serious issue for pathologists. To identify its cause, I visited the X-ray room to watch how the postoperative radiography was being conducted. At that time, late Dr. Ohashi was inserting a catheter into the main pancreatic duct for radiography. He was repeating radiography from multiple directions to allow the direction of main pancreatic duct to be imaged as clearly as possible. I learned that while the postoperative radiograms became clearer, the resected specimen was damaged more severely, making histological examination extremely difficult. Thus, it is important to handle the specimen in such a way as to avoid self-lysis. Because postoperative radiography is performed using Urografin diluted with physiological saline, I asked Dr. Ohashi to use formalin instead of physiological saline for diluting Urografin. As a result, specimens without self-lysis became available for histological examination. To further facilitate preparation of autolysis-free histological specimens, contrast material diluted with formalin began to be infused via the artery supplying the pancreas and via the common bile duct during postoperative radiography, and a standard method for handling postoperative specimens became established. In most of the IPMN cases presented in this atlas, the specimens were handled in this method, resulting in preservation of a clear papillary structure even in cases with papillary lesions of great height, as readers can readily see.

Improvement in diagnostic imaging of pancreas can be achieved by comparing preoperative images, postoperative images and histological findings in each case and by sufficient analysis as to which histological findings support which changes in the images. Discussions between clinicians and pathologists until full consensus can be reached are important for this purpose. This atlas is a collection of IPMN images and histological findings, serving as the basis for such discussions. I hope it will become useful for facilitated diagnosis in routine clinical practice.

Introduction

In 1982, Ohashi and Takagi et al. of our hospital adopted the name "mucus-producing pancreatic cancer" to indicate a type of pancreatic cancer that was characterized clinically by diffuse dilatation of the main pancreatic duct, marked enlargement of the opening of the duodenal papilla and discharge of a large amount of mucus from this area, reporting it as a pancreatic cancer with a relatively good prognosis[1]. Furthermore, on the basis of the ERCP findings, they proposed a new classification of pancreatic cancer, dividing it into types I through IV on the basis of the anatomical relationship between the pancreatic cancer and the main pancreatic duct[2]. The "mucus-producing pancreatic cancer" mentioned above was positioned as type III, and this disease began to be called "Cancer Institute type III" pancreatic cancer. Later, as the number of surgically treated cases of this cancer increased, it was revealed that among the cases of this cancer presenting with similar clinical features, there were cases in which the lesions were primarily located within the main pancreatic duct, cases with the lesions additionally found in the branches of the pancreatic duct and also cases with the lesions covering the pancreatic duct branches to the main pancreatic duct. It was also revealed that there were many cases in which distinction between cancer and adenoma was difficult. As a result, the term "mucus-producing pancreatic tumor" began to be used to indicate these cancers and adenomas collectively. Later, Yanagisawa et al. adopted the term "pancreatic duct-dilated-type mucinous cystadenoma" to indicate lesions developing like bronchiectasis-like lesions in the pancreatic duct branches without manifesting the characteristic clinical signs of "mucus-producing pancreatic tumor," and proposed it as a branch-affecting type of disease entity[3-5]. Subsequently, the concept of "mucus-producing pancreatic tumor" was merged with the above-mentioned "pancreatic duct-dilated-type of mucinous cystadenoma" to yield the histological concept of "intraductal papillary tumor." In Japan, this disease concept was adopted as "intraductal papillary mucinous tumor of the pancreas" in the General Rules for Surgical and Pathological Studies on Pancreatic Cancer. It also spread rapidly on a global scale, resulting in its adoption in the WHO histological classification of tumours of the exocrine pancreas as "intraductal papillary-mucinous tumour (IPMT)"[4]. This tumor, initially called "mucus-producing pancreatic tumor" because of its characteristic clinical feature of producing large amounts of mucus ("high mucus-producing potential"), is histologically viewed as "intraductal papillary mucinous tumor (IPMT)"[6]. Clinically, patients with IPMT lacking the "high mucus-producing potential" are also seen sometimes. For these reasons, this disease came to be called IPMT (a histological disease entity). At present, the term "intraductal papillary-mucinous neoplasm (IPMN)" is used across the world[6,7] and the important concept of exocrine pancreatic tumors as compared to invasive pancreatic duct cancer is well known. Histologically, it is additionally known that borderline lesions between IPMN and mucinous cystic neoplasm (MCN) or pancreatic intraepithelial neoplasia (PanIN)[8] are not uncommon, over which question, there has been much debate. If the relationship among these 3 lesions can be clarified by molecular-biological methods[9], it is highly probable that the mechanism underlying the onset of pancreatic tumors, and eventually pancreatic cancer, will come to be elucidated.

A quarter of a century has already passed since the entity was first proposed by Ohashi and Takagi et al. During this period, numerous cases of IPMN treated by surgical resection, not only in Japan, but also at many facilities across the world, have been reported. Thanks to accumulation of data from many resected cases and advances in the precision of diagnostic imaging modalities, it seems that the indications of surgery in cases of IPMN have been changing gradually, not only at the Cancer Institute but also at many other facilities. The authors have been keenly aware of the necessity of reviewing the cases of IPMN resected surgically at our hospital and summarizing their data for utilization in future diagnosis and treatment of this disease. Now, we have summarized all surgically resected cases of IPMN at the Cancer

Institute and are presenting the findings in the form of this atlas, focusing on the cases of cancer. It would be our great pleasure if this book does not end as a simple collection of cases, but serves as a source of clues to readers when discussing appropriate diagnosis and treatment of IPMN.

Authors

References

1) Ohashi K, Murakami Y, Maruyama M, et al : Four case of mucus-producing pancreatic cancer—Focusing on specific findings from the duodenal papilla. Progress of Digestive Endoscopy **20** : 348-351, 1982.
2) Ohashi K, Maruyama M, Yokoyama Y, et al : New classification of ERCP findings of pancreatic cancer. Gastroenterology **80** : 1241, 1981.
3) Yanagisawa A, Kato Y, Sugano H, et al : Pathology of pancreatic cyst—Classification of cystic lesions including atypical epithelium. Tan to Sui **5** : 1079-1085, 1984.
4) Yanagisawa A, Ohashi K, Hori M, et al : Ductectatic-type mucinous cystadenoma and cystadenocarcinoma of thehuman pancreas : a novel clinicopathological entity. Jpn J Cancer Res **84** : 474-479, 1993.
5) Itai Y, Ohashi K, Nagai H, et al : =Ductectatic@mucinous cystadenoma and cystadenocarcinoma of the pancreas. Radiology **161** : 697-700, 1986.
6) Longnecker DS, Hruban RH, Adler G, et al : Intraductal papillary-mucinous neoplasms of the pancreas. In : Hamilton SR, Aaltonen LA (eds) World Health Organization classification of tumours. Pathlogy & genetics. Tumours of the digestive system. Lyon : IARC Press, **2000** : 237-240.
7) Hruban RH, PitmanMB, Klimstra DS : Tumors of the pancreas. In : AFIP Atlas of Tumor Pathology. Fourth series, Fascicle 6. Washington DC : American Registry of Pathology, **2007** : 75-110.
8) Hruban RH, Takaori K, Klimstra DS, et al : An illustrated consensus on the classification of pancreatic intraepithelial neoplasia and intraductal papillary mucinous neoplasms. Am J Surg Pathol **28** : 977-987, 2004.
9) Yanagisawa A, Kato Y, Ohtake K, et al : c-Ki-ras point mutation in ductectatic-type mucinous cystic neoplasm ofthe pancreas. Jpn J Cancer Res **82** : 1057-1060, 1991.

Acknowledgments

I felt as if it were a "wave" directed at pancreatic cancer when I witnessed the scene at the Cancer Institute which I joined in the early half of the 1980s. There were many physicians taking upon them the challenge of early diagnosis and early treatment of pancreatic cancer, beyond the borders of specialties. Now, nearly three decades later, pancreatic cancer still remains one of the most intractable of cancers among gastrointestinal cancers. Amidst such a wave, in 1982 Dr. Kazuhiko Ohashi et al. proposed the disease entity of "mucus-producing pancreatic cancer"[1]. In 1984, "Illustrations for Early Diagnosis of Pancreatic Cancer" was published by Dr. Kunio Takagi et al.[2]. In those days, the staff of the Internal Medicine Department waiting in the operating room (e. g., Dr. Kazuhiko Ohashi and Dr. Yoshifumi Murakami) performed radiography of the resected specimens immediately after the resection carried out by the surgical staff such as Dr. Tamaki Kajitani, Dr. Kunio Takagi and Dr. Masaharu Hori. Several days later, full-section pathological specimens (5- to 8 mm) were prepared from the fixed specimens in a direction perpendicular to the main pancreatic duct to enable easy comparison with the preoperative CT findings. With reference to the macroscopic features of the sectional plane and the findings from radiography, the anatomical location of tumors "in and around the main pancreatic duct" was clarified, and through comparison with the preoperative images, physicians from different specialties debated about the preoperatively anticipated development diagrams and reviewed the preoperative diagnosis. Then, on a later day, the preoperative images were reviewed again for reflecting on the preoperative judgments while referring to the histopathological findings. This sequence of steps was the "wave" towards the goal of approaching the "real" lesions through cooperation among surgeons, internists, radiologists and pathologists. The author was within this wave and repeatedly diagnosed and treated this disease, with subsequent reflection, following the course of the above-mentioned senior physicians. What we have done in this atlas is nothing more than putting in order the data from numerous cases of IPMN accumulated until date at the Cancer Institute. It is a great honor for us to publish this atlas. We would like to express our sincere gratitude not only to the above-listed senior physicians, but also to many of our other senior colleagues and junior physicians who are working actively across Japan, for their cooperation in the editing of this book. Direct guidance about the diagnosis and treatment of not only "mucus-producing pancreatic cancer," but also of pancreatic cancer in general, was provided by my teachers Dr. Kunio Takagi and Dr. Masaharu Hori. Dr. Takagi used to take the author to the endoscopy room soon after a specimen of IPMN was removed, where they inserted an electronic scope into the dilated resected specimen and washed out the mucus, followed by spraying of indigo carmine, to show us the intraductal papillary tumor. Pictures taken at these times have also been adopted in this book, with some of them also adopted in the General Rules for Surgical and Pathological Studies on Pancreatic Cancer[3]. Even at present, I can vividly remember the surprise I experienced when viewing the fantastic close-up image of the tumor on the video monitor.

I also owe much also to Dr. Yo Kato (Cancer Institute), who was always willing, even if he was busy, to take me to the Discussion Microscope and give me precise guidance every time I consulted him about any difficulties I faced during histopathological diagnosis of "mucus-producing pancreatic cancer". I can proudly say that each case adopted in this atlas (mentioned later) was checked by Dr. Kato. Furthermore, I would like to express my deep gratitude to the staff of the department of pathology for their cooperation and support as coworkers, as well as to the pathological technologists who prepared the full-section specimens, always nicely.

We also received much cooperation from the radiologic technologists who were willing to cooperate during the sample radiographing, even at late hours of the day, and from four members of the photography office (Mr. Katsumi Takano, Mr. Kazuo Sanuga, Mr. Shigeharu Kato and Mr. Jun Takano) in connection with the adoption of images and photographs for this atlas. I would also like to express my deep appreciation for these people.

Department of Surgery, Mitaka Center Hospital

Makoto Seki

References

1) Ohashi K, Murakami Y, Maruyama M, et al : Four cases of mucus-producing pancreatic cancer—Focusing on specific findings from the duodenal papilla. Progress of Digestive Endoscopy **20** : 348-351, 1982.
2) Takagi K, Takekoshi T, Maruyama M, et al : Illustrations for early diagnosis of pancreatic cancer, Igaku Shoin, Tokyo, 1984.
3) Japan Pancreas Society : General Rules for Surgical and Pathological Studies on Pancreatic Cancer, 5th edition, Kanehara Shuppan, Tokyo, 2002

Contents

Preface

Recommendation ·· Haruo Sugano   i

Recommendation ·· Yuji Nimura   iii

Forward ·· Kunio Takagi   v

Upon publication of this book ····································· Akio Yanagisawa   vii

Introduction ·· Authors   ix

Acknowledgments ·· Makoto Seki   xi

I. Dawn of "mucus-producing pancreatic cancer" and its transition—until intraductal papillary mucinous neoplasm (IPMN) ······················ 1

II. Clinicopathologic Findings in Cases of IPMN treated by Resection ············ 6

Case 1 Relatively typical main-pancreatic duct type intraductal papillary-mucinous carcinoma (IPMC) without pancreatic duct invasion that required distinction from the mixed-type ································ 16

Case 2 Invasive cancer of pancreatic tail intraductal papillary-mucinous neoplasm (IPMN) origin presenting with typical signs of mucinous carcinoma ··· 25

Case 3 Mixed-type non-invasive intraductal papillary-mucinous carcinoma (IPMC) of the pancreatic body spreading widely within a secondary branch of the pancreatic duct ·· 34

Case 4 Minimally invasive mixed-type of intraductal papillary-mucinous carcinoma (IPMC) of the pancreatic body without macroscopically detectable intramural nodule ··· 43

Case 5 Branch duct-type non-invasive intraductal papillary-mucinous carcinoma (IPMC) with concurrent carcinoma in situ (CIS) at three sites ······· 52

Case 6　Invasive carcinoma derived from branch-duct type intraductal papillary-mucinous neoplasm (IPMN): A case with inferred transition to invasive carcinoma during a 5-year follow-up course ······································61

Case 7　Main-duct type intraductal papillary-mucinous adenoma (IPMA) showing typical morphologic features ···72

Case 8　Typical intraductal papillary-mucinous adenoma (IPMA), with severe atypia, of the head of the pancreas, in which an intraductal lesion was noted in the main pancreatic duct on examination of the resected specimen by fiberoptic endoscopy ···81

Case 9　A large moderately atypical intraductal papillary-mucinous adenoma (IPMA) measuring 5 cm in maximum diameter with a mural nodule ·······90

Case 10　Non-invasive intraductal papillary-mucinous carcinoma (IPMC) spreading across the entire pancreas ···100

I. Dawn of "mucus-producing pancreatic cancer" and its transition—until intraductal papillary mucinous neoplasm (IPMN)

1. Background for proposing the concept of mucus-producing pancreatic cancer

In 1982, we reported 4 cases of "mucus-producing pancreatic cancer" from our hospital[1], following which we encountered cases of pancreatic tumors that resembled mucus-producing cancer, but were histologically rated as benign adenomas. From these cases, the concept of "mucus-producing pancreatic tumor" was born, encompassing both cancer and adenoma. Subsequently, "mucus-producing pancreatic neoplasm" in which excessive mucus production (a clinical feature of "mucus-producing pancreatic tumor") was not seen were found, which led to unification of the concepts into a histological disease entity called "intraductal papillary neoplasm of pancreas." This disease concept has been adopted as "intraductal papillary-mucinous neoplasm" in the Classification of Pancreatic Carcinoma in Japan[2]. The concept has also spread rapidly overseas, resulting in listing of "Intraductal papillary-mucinous neoplasm (IPMN)" as one category of the World Health Organization (WHO) Classification of Exocrine Pancreatic Tumors[3]. IPMN is now divided into two types:

1) Intraductal papillary-mucinous carcinoma (IPMC)
2) Intraductal papillary-mucinous adenoma (IPMA)

We consider it necessary to record the first reports of this disease which has now come to be recognized around the world. Of the various features of "mucus-producing pancreatic cancer," enlargement of the opening of the duodenal papilla is one of the most striking features. The finding shown in the right column of Fig. 1, i. e. enlarged opening of duodenal papilla showing viscous mucus discharge, is quite impressive as compared to the appearance of the normal papilla shown in the left column of the same figure; once seen, it is difficult to forget. Fig. 2 shows a pancreatogram of the resected specimen in this case after pancreatectomy, which shows signs of tumor at two sites of the diffusely dilated main pancreatic duct (one in the pancreatic head region and the other in the pancreatic body region). Histologically, the cancer was rated as non-invasive early cancer confined to the main pancreatic duct. Pooling of viscous gelatin-like mucus was noted in the dilated main pancreatic duct.

Table 1 shows the year of diagnosis, the surgical procedure (extent of spread) and the outcomes of the 4 cases of "mucus-producing pancreatic cancer" reported in 1981 at the Kanto Bloc Meeting of the Japan Gastroenterological Endoscopy Society and then published in a paper in 1982[1]. Figures 3 and 4 graphically represent the papillary findings,

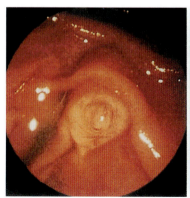
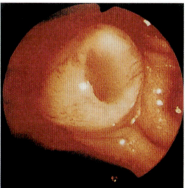

Fig. 1 Mucus-producing pancreatic cancer (enlarged opening of the duodenal papilla)

Normal papilla   Enlarged papillary opening

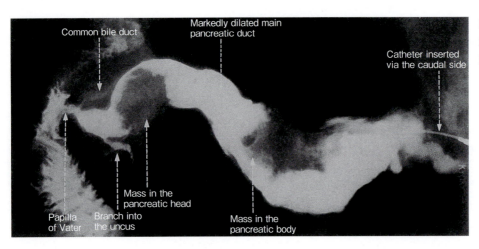

Fig. 2 Pancreatography of the resected entire pancreas (Case 2)

Table 1 Years of diagnosis and the outcomes in the 4 cases of mucus-producing pancreatic cancer

Operation date		Surgical procedure	Outcomes
Case 1 age 70 female May 6, 1979		Pancreatoduodenectomy (early cancer)	Death after 12 years 9 months (myocardial infarction)
	[8 months]		
Case 2 age 62 male Jan 23, 1980		Total pancreatectomy (early cancer)	Death after 10 years 4 months (debility)
	[7 months]		
Case 3 age 63 male Aug 27, 1980		Distal pancreatectomy (early cancer)	Death after 6 years 1 month (metachronous pancreatic head cancer)
	[11 months]		
Case 4 age 77 male Jul 10, 1981		Total pancreatectomy (advanced cancer)	Death after 2 months (cancer)

Report at a professional society meeting on Dec 12, 1981 (2 years 6 months after Case 1 was encountered)

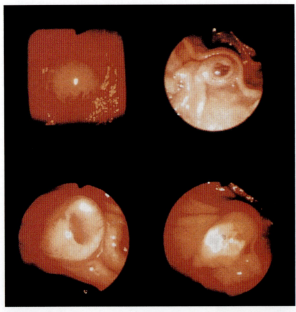

Fig. 3 Papilla in 4 cases of mucus-producing pancreatic cancer

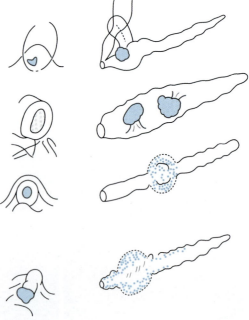

Fig. 4 Lesions in 4 cases of mucus-producing pancreatic cancer

the changes in the main pancreatic duct and the findings related to the lesions in each case.

In the first case, the patient had undergone external cholecystostomy because of jaundice[4]. Endoscopic retrograde cholangiopancreatography (ERCP) revealed swelling of the duodenal papilla and enlargement of the papilla opening, however, there was no mucus discharge (Fig. 3, upper left). Macroscopic observation of sections of the tissue specimen resected by pancreatoduodenectomy revealed a dilated main pancreatic duct and a cystic lesion in the pancreatic head, with gelatin-like mucus filling the cyst, and partial formation of a fistula between the common bile duct and pancreatic duct (Fig. 4, uppermost). A diagnosis of intraductal cancer was made based on the macroscopic findings. The lesion was pathologically diagnosed at first as a benign ductal cyst. However, Dr. Kunio Ohta, Head of our Pathology department, made the final diagnosis of cystadenocarinoma on the grounds that few cellular components were seen in the mucus.

The second case[5] was encountered 8 months after the first. Endoscopic examination in this case showed swelling of the duodenal papilla, with marked dilatation of the papillary orifice discharging viscous pancreatic fluid (Fig. 1, right ; Fig. 3, lower left). After endoscopic incision of the duodenal papilla, a small-diameter endoscope (GIP-P2) was inserted into the main pancreatic duct for observation and biopsy of the tumor. The tumor was diagnosed as a papillary adenocarcinoma based on the histological findings. Macroscopic examination of the cut surface along the major axis of the entire resected pancreas revealed two relatively large papillary tumors (one in the pancreatic head region and the other in the pancreatic body region) within the segment of the main pancreatic duct that showed marked diffuse dilatation, and the main pancreatic duct was filled with gelatin-like discharge (Fig. 2). The conventionally well-known pattern of main pancreatic duct dilatation arises from stenosis of the main pancreatic duct due to pancreatic cancer or pancreatitis, which causes dilatation of the caudal segment of the pancreatic duct. In this case, however, the main pancreatic duct showed <u>diffuse dilatation without accompanying stenosis</u>, which had not been recognized previously. This seemed to be a previously unknown condition in which pooling of the entire main pancreatic duct with viscous mucus secreted from the pancreatic cancer caused diffuse dilatation of the main pancreatic duct. Although pancreatic ductal cancer has conventionally been considered to arise from the pancreatic duct branches in many cases, the cancer in this case seemed to arise from the main pancreatic duct itself, the diameter of which in the absence of dilatation was 4-5 mm at the maximum. Thus, this was <u>evidently a case of carcinoma developing in the main pancreatic duct</u>. These new findings, found in abundance, were quite surprising. We intuitively felt that the lesion in this second case resembled that in the first case.

The third case[6] was encountered 7 months after the second. In this case, endoscopy revealed marked enlargement of the opening of the duodenal papilla and discharge of viscous mucus from the orifice of the papilla (Fig. 3, upper right). At this point of time, we performed pancreatography, bearing in mind the papillary findings of the second case. Cystiform dilatation of the main pancreatic duct was noted in the pancreatic body region, based on which we judged that this area was affected by pancreatic cancer.

We were very lucky to encounter these 3 cases, one case after another, during the relatively short period of 7 or 8 months.

In 1982, Dr. Kazuhiko Ohashi proposed the concept of "mucus-producing pancreatic cancer" for the first time in the world, reporting 4 cases presenting with clinical features akin to those mentioned above. In his personal communication to Dr. Kunio Takagi, Dr. Ohashi reviewed those days, stating : "When I saw the first case, I did not recognize it as a new condition. When I saw the second case, I got the impression that it resembled the first case, but I still did not understand the value of the case. On seeing a third similar case, I began to consider that the lesion may represent a new disease concept. Thus, three cases had to be seen before I could start recognizing the novelty of this condition. Such a process is also experienced in the discovery of other new events, isn't it?" Dr. Ohashi additionally stated the following in "The fifteen years of 'so-called mucus-producing pancreatic cancer' viewed by the proponent of this disease concept"[17] : "The

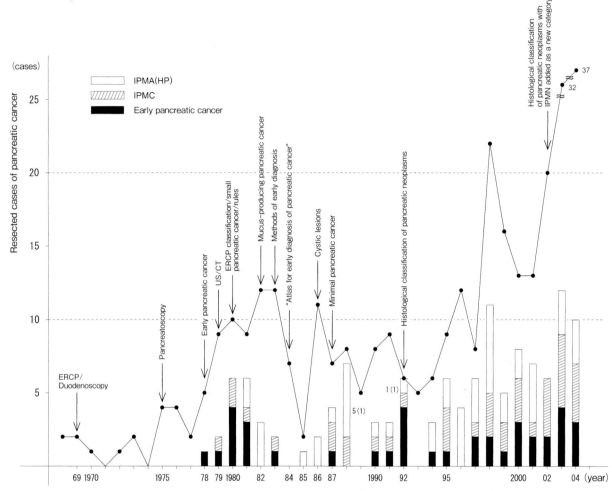

Fig. 5 Annual course of early diagnosis and treatment of pancreatic cancer (Cancer Institute, 1969-2004)

expression 'mucus-producing pancreatic cancer' was adopted simply because excretion of mucus from the papillary opening was the most striking clinical feature." He concluded the statement by saying that proposal of this disease as a new entity was made under the background of the efforts for early diagnosis of pancreatic cancer made jointly in those days by the Cancer Institute Hospital (Departments of Internal Medicine, Surgery and Radiology) and the Cancer Institute (Department of Pathology)[7].

2. How was mucus-producing pancreatic cancer discovered?

In regard to the question of how "mucus-producing pancreatic cancer" was discovered, Fig. 5 seems to contain the key answer to "How?" This figure graphically represents the history of early diagnosis and treatment of pancreatic cancer at the Cancer Institute Hospital as well as the annual numbers of patients undergoing resection of pancreatic cancer and their clinical data between the years 1969 and 2004. After the successful introduction of ERCP in 1969[8], efforts were concentrated on the diagnosis of pancreatic cancer (particularly early diagnosis) by ERCP, but during the 9-year period until 1977, only 2 cases of pancreatic cancer per year, on average, were treated by resection. In 1978, however, early-stage pancreatic head cancer without jaundice was detected for the first time by ERCP after an elevated urinary amylase level was detected and the cancer was resected successfully[9]. Also, in some cases, elevated serum or urinary amylase levels, suggestive of pancreatitis accompanying the pancreatic cancer, led to early diagnosis of the pancreatic cancer[10]. Thus, the practice of proactively performing ERCP in patients found to have elevated amylase levels began to be adopted

Table 2 Frequency of four types of pancreatic cancer (early cancer, advanced cancer, IPMC and IPMA) during each 5-year period (some duplications of early cancer and IPMC)

Period	1978-1982	1938-1987	1988-1992	1993-1997	1998-2002	2003-2004	Total
Early cancer	9	2	6	4	10	7	38
	(IPMC 3)	(IPMC 2)	(IPMC 4)	(IPMC 2)	(IPMC 7)	(IPMC 5)	(IPMC 23)
Advanced cancer	30	32	21	23	54	52	212
IPMC	4	3	5	4	13	9	38
	(Invasive 1)	(Invasive 1)	(Invasive 1)	(Invasive 2)	(Invasive 6)	(Invasive 4)	(Invasive 15)
IPMA	5	4	8	11	14	6	48
Total	45	39	36	40	84	69	313

IPMC : Intraductal papillary-mucinous carcinoma, IPMA : Intraductal papillary-mucinous adenoma

in 1978. Since then, the annual number of surgically resected cases of pancreatic cancer rose from year to year, with 33 cases treated by resection during the 4-year period until 1981. These cases included the 4 cases of "mucus-producing pancreatic cancer." Thus, experience of many cases of resected pancreatic cancer within a short period of time may be one answer to the question of "How was mucus-producing pancreatic cancer discovered?" There is another possible answer. In cases of solid pancreatic cancer, pancreatic duct stenosis caused by the tumor (organic stenosis) led to the diagnosis of accompanying pancreatitis. In cases of "mucus-producing pancreatic cancer," however, the stenosis was not organic, but functional (due to viscous mucus produced by the tumor), and resulted in accompanying pancreatitis (elevated amylase level, extragastric compression, and pancreatic duct dilatation). Two of the 4 cases with "mucus-producing pancreatic cancer" showed elevated urinary amylase levels and signs of extragastric compression and were found to have lesions on ERCP.

We may therefore say that the presence of "mucus-producing pancreatic cancer" was revealed as a byproduct of many efforts made for early diagnosis of pancreatic cancer primarily using ERCP, rather than as an outcome of any work intended at discovery of "mucus-producing pancreatic cancer."

3. Transition from mucus-producing pancreatic cancer to IPMN

As described above, the term "mucus-producing pancreatic cancer" was later modified into "mucus-producing pancreatic neoplasm" encompassing benign tumors, followed by changes into terms including cases free of clinical signs of excessive mucus production (i. e., tumors without high mucus-producing potential), i. e. "intraductal papillary neoplasm" →intraductal papillary-mucinous tumor (IPMT)→IPMN. If early pancreatic cancer is defined as "pancreatic cancer confined to the pancreas, regardless of the tumor size, i. e., [s (−), rp (−), n (−)] pancreatic cancer" as described in references[1,2], needless to say, many tumors of the IPMC category will fall under the definition of early pancreatic cancer.

Fig. 5 shows a bar graph of the numbers of cases with early pancreatic cancer (■), IPMC (▨) and IPMA (□) (some duplications of early pancreatic cancer and IPMC). At our hospital, the first case of early pancreatic cancer was encountered in 1978 and the first case of IPMC in 1979. Thereafter, one or two cases of each of these tumors have been encountered annually, without any sharp increase in the number of cases. From 1997 onward, however, the number of cases with these tumors has been tending to rise evidently. A similar course was also followed for benign IPMN (IPMA), with 1 or 2 cases recorded per year from 1981 (2 cases) to 1995 and a slight increase to about 2-4 cases per year from 1996 onwards. The number of cases with each of these three kinds of tumor has been showing a similar upward trend since 1996 or 1997, probably influenced most by the rapid spread of screening by diagnostic imaging modalities (ultrasonography [US] and computed tomography [CT]) in Japan during this period.

Table 2 summarizes the course of changes after 1978 divided into five-year periods. A sharp rise in the number of cases began to be seen in 1998 for early pancreatic cancer and IPMC and in 1988 for IPMA.

II. Clinicopathologic Findings in Cases of IPMN treated by Resection

1. Subjects and Methods

The study population consisted of 82 patients with intraductal papillary mucinous neoplasm (IPMN) treated by resection of the tumor collected during the 26-year period from 1979 to 2004. The sex ratio was 52 : 30 (male to female), and the mean age was 66.4 years. Each formalin-fixed resected specimen was cut stepwise in sections measuring 5-8 mm in thickness, as much at right angles to the course of the main pancreatic duct as possible (serial crosswise sections), while referring to cholangiopancreatograms of the resected specimen, whereby the tumor diameter was measured accurately. The intraductal maximum diameter of the lesion was recorded, irrespective of whether the lesion was diagnosed by histopathology as being benign or malignant.

In lesions showing histopathologic continuity of the IPMN with the surrounding regions invaded by the tumor, the remaining intraductal tumor region after supposed resection of the invaded regions, was defined here as an independent entity for the diagnostic differentiation of IPMN-derived invasive carcinoma from ordinary-type invasive pancreatic ductal carcinoma. Among the IPMN-derived invasive carcinomas, there was a group in which the extent of tumor invasion was only slight, with the tumor protruding only slightly beyond the pancreatic duct wall- the carcinoma was confined to the pancreas and there was no evidence of lymph node metastasis ; the prognosis in these cases was as favorable as that in cases of non-invasive carcinoma ; these lesions were dealt with separately as minimally invasive in this study. Thus, the histologic diagnosis of IPMN was made according to the following classification in order of increasing atypia and malignancy : hyperplasia, adenoma, non-invasive carcinoma, minimally invasive carcinoma, and invasive carcinoma.

As for IPMN lesions, the primary tumor was within the main pancreatic duct lumen or stretched over the main pancreatic duct and branch ducts or was confined to a pancreatic duct branch. The tumors were classified as the main pancreatic duct type, mixed type or the branch type, and the clinicopathological data were analyzed by the type and size of the tumors.

2. Results

1) Clinical findings of IPMN

①Clinical breakdown of the IPMN cases

The sites of tumor location in the pancreas are shown in Table 1. The distribution of the tumor sites did not appear to be substantially different from that of usual invasive carcinoma of the pancreatic duct, but the tumor involved the entire pancreas in 5 patients (6%). When classified according to primary site of the tumor in the pancreatic duct, there were 12 patients with main pancreatic duct-type lesions, 16 patients with mixed-type lesions, and 54 patients with branch-type lesions.

②Clues to the diagnosis of IPMN (Table 2)

Clues to the diagnosis of IPMN are summarized in Table 2 ; however, it would be somewhat problematic to deal with

Table 1 Sites of tumor location

Site of tumor location	No. of patients
Head	42
Head to body	7
Body	19
Body to tail	8
Tail	1
Whole pancreas	5
Total	82

Table 2 Clues to diagnosis of the tumor

Symptomatic (35)		
	Upper abdominal pain	25
	Back pain	3
	Diabetes exacerbation	2
	Jaundice	2
	Impaired appetite	2
	Melena	1
Asymptomatic (47)		
	Abdominal US	32
	Abdominal CT	12
	Serum amylase elevation	2
	CA19-9 elevation	1

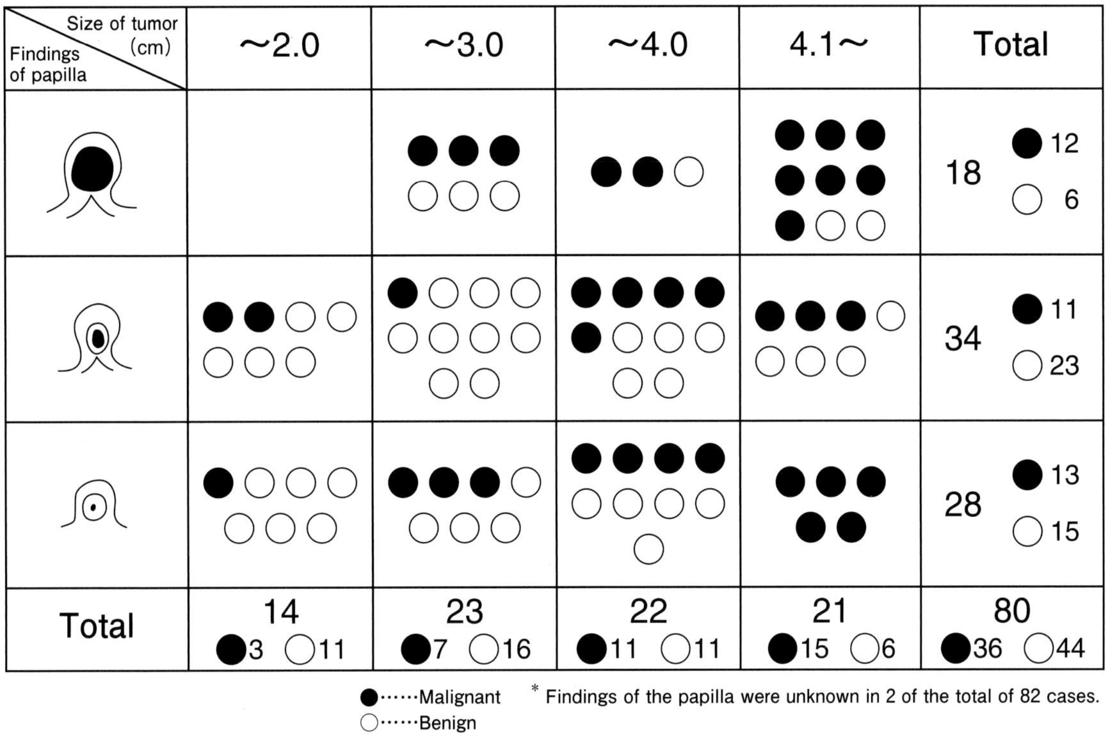

● ……Malignant   ○ ……Benign   *Findings of the papilla were unknown in 2 of the total of 82 cases.

Fig. 1 Relationships of the macroscopic findings of the duodenal papilla with the tumor size and benign/malignant nature of the tumor

the clues to the diagnosis in the early phase and late phase of the study together, as this retrospective investigation covered a long period : screening and diagnostic imaging devices and techniques have advanced over the years, with an increase in the rate of diagnosis of IPMN even in the absence of symptoms. As seen in Table 2, 35 of the 82 patients had some of the symptom (s) and the remaining 47 patients were asymptomatic. Upper abdominal pain was the most frequent symptom among the symptomatic patients, whereas among the asymptomatic patients, initial discovery of the lesions by ultrasonography (US)/computed tomography (CT) was overwhelmingly more frequent than diagnosis by other imaging modalities.

③**Macroscopic findings of the duodenal papilla** (Fig. 1)

In general, in cases of IPMN, viscous mucous fluid produced by the tumor stagnates in the pancreatic duct, frequently causing dilatation of the pancreatic duct and of the duodenal papillary orifice, and excretion of the viscous mucous fluid

Table 3 Relationship between the diameter of the main pancreatic duct and benign/malignant nature of the tumor

Diameter of the main pancreatic duct (mm)	~3	~7	~11	12~
Main pancreatic-duct type	0	1 (1)	4 (3)	7 (7)
Mixed type	0	6 (3)	3 (2)	8 (7)
Branch type	6 (0)	34 (9)	11 (5)	2 (1)
Total (No. of carcinoma cases)	6 (0)	41 (13)	18 (10)	17 (15)

from the papillary orifice. Figure 1 illustrates the correlations between the findings of the duodenal papilla and the size and benign nature/malignant nature of the tumors. These correlations are considered to vary with the location of the primary tumor, that is, whether the primary tumor is a main pancreatic-duct type, mixed-type or branch-type tumor. In general, in the presence of a wide opening of the papilla of Vater, the tumor tended to be malignant (it was cancerous in 12 (67%) of the 18 patients with widening of the duodenal papilla). Even in cases without widening of the duodenal papilla (5 cases), the tumor tended to be malignant in cases where the lesion measured >4 cm in diameter. The tumor in these 5 patients was advanced, with the tumor filling the dilated pancreatic duct, possibly being already past the phase of viscous mucous fluid excretion through a widened papilla.

④**Relationship between the diameter of the main pancreatic duct and benign/malignant nature of the tumor** (Table 3)

In cases of IPMN, it is common for the tumor-produced mucous fluid to stagnate in the pancreatic duct causing dilatation of the main pancreatic duct, irrespective of whether the tumor is of the main pancreatic-duct type, mixed-type or branch-type. It is necessary to indicate the diameter of the main pancreatic duct for each tumor type, since the diameter is strongly influenced by the primary site of the tumor (Table 3). When the relationship of the main pancreatic duct diameter with the benign/malignant nature of the tumor was assessed for each tumor type, the frequency of malignancy in patients with a main duct diameter of >7 mm was 91% (10/11) for cases with main pancreatic-duct type tumors, 82% (9/11) for cases with mixed-type tumors, and 46% (6/13) for cases with branch-type tumors ; thus, the lesions in cases with a tumor diameter of the pancreatic duct of >7 mm tended to be malignant. Overall, the frequency of malignancy in cases with a main pancreatic duct diameter of >7 mm was 71% (25/35) and the frequency of malignancy in cases with a main duct diameter ≧12 mm was 88% (15/17). Thus, the physician/surgeon should bear in mind that these tumors have high mucus-producing potential and that the likelihood of malignancy is high in patients in whom the main pancreatic duct measures >7 mm in diameter.

2) Surgical pathologic findings of IPMN

①**Histological breakdown of IPMNs by the site of tumor location** (Table 4)

The 82 cases of IPMN were classified according to the site of tumor location in the pancreatic duct into 12 cases of main pancreatic-duct type tumors, 17 cases of mixed-type tumors, and 53 cases of branch-type tumors. The frequency of cancer was 92% (11/12) in main pancreatic-duct type tumors, 71% (12/17) in mixed-type tumors and 28% (15/53) in branch-type tumors ; it tended to be considerably lower in branch-type tumors as compared to that in pancreatic duct-type and mixed-type tumors. The frequency of invasive carcinoma case was 45% (5/11) in main pancreatic-duct type tumors, 58% (7/12) in mixed-type tumors, and 27% (4/15) in branch-type tumors. The frequency of invasive carcinoma among all cases of malignant IPMN was highest for mixed-type tumors, followed, in order by main pancreatic duct-type tumors and branch-type tumors, although the differences among the three types were not significant.

Table 4 Histological breakdown of IPMNs by the site of tumor location (Cancer Institute, 1979 to 2004)

Tumor location	Histologic type	No. of patients	%
Main pancreatic-duct type	Hyperplasia	0	0
	Adenoma	1	8.3
	Carcinoma		
	Non-invasive	5 ⎤	
	Minimally invasive	1 ⎬ 11	91.7
	Invasive	5 ⎦	
	Total	12	100
Mixed type	Hyperplasia	0	0
	Adenoma	5	29.4
	Carcinoma		
	Non-invasive	4 ⎤	
	Minimally invasive	1 ⎬ 12	70.6
	Invasive	7 ⎦	
	Total	17	100
Branch type	Hyperplasia	2	3.8
	Adenoma	36	67.9
	Carcinoma		
	Non-invasive	8 ⎤	
	Minimally invasive	3 ⎬ 15	28.3
	Invasive	4 ⎦	
	Total	53	100

②**Histological breakdown of main pancreatic-duct type and mixed-type IPMNs by the tumor size** (Table 5)

The frequency of malignancy was high, irrespective of the tumor size in the combined main pancreatic-duct type (12 cases) and mixed-type (17 cases) tumors (29 cases in total). Among the 17 cases with a tumor size of >4 cm, a high percentage (65%；11/17) had invasive carcinoma. However, there was one case of invasive carcinoma among the tumors measuring less than 2 cm in diameter.

③**Histological breakdown of branch-type IPMNs by the tumor size** (Table 6)

Of the 53 cases of branch-type IPMNs, the frequency of cancer classified by the tumor size was as follows：9% (1/11)

Table 5 Histological breakdown of main pancreatic-duct type and mixed-type IPMNs by the tumor size (Cancer Institute, 1979 to 2004)

Histologic type	Size (mm)*			
	~20	~30	~40	41~
Adenoma	1 (33%)	1 (33%)	2 (33%)	2 (12%)
Carcinoma				
Non-invasive	1 ⎫	1 ⎫	1 ⎫	3 ⎫
Minimally invasive	0 ⎬ 2 (67%)	0 ⎬ 2 (67%)	0 ⎬ 4 (67%)	1 ⎬ 15 (88%)
Invasive	1 ⎭	1 ⎭	3 ⎭	11 ⎭
Total	3 (100%)	3 (100%)	6 (100%)	17 (100%)

*Maximum diameter of intraductal spread

Table 6 Histological breakdown of branch-type IPMNs by the tumor size (Cancer Institute, 1979 to 2004)

Histologic type	Size (mm)*			
	~20	~30	~40	41~
Hyperplasia	1 (9%)	1 (5%)	0	0
Adenoma	9 (82%)	14 (66%)	8 (50%)	5 (100%)
Carcinoma				
Non-invasive	1 ⎫	3 ⎫	4 ⎫	0 ⎫
Minimally invasive	0 ⎬ 1 (9%)	1 ⎬ 6 (29%)	2 ⎬ 8 (50%)	0 ⎬ 0 (0%)
Invasive	0 ⎭	2 ⎭	2 ⎭	0 ⎭
Total	11 (100%)	21 (100%)	16 (100%)	5 (100%)

*Maximum diameter of intraductal spread

for tumors measuring ≤2 cm in diameter, 29% (6/21) for tumors measuring 2 to 3 cm in diameter, and 50% (8/16) for tumors measuring 3 to 4 cm in diameter ; on the other hand, there were no cases of cancer among the 5 tumors measuring >4 cm in diameter. Nevertheless, a high degree grade of histologic atypia, representing borderline cases, was seen in 2 of 5 cases of adenoma exceeding 4 cm in diameter. Thus, cancer was found at a relatively high frequency in tumors measuring >3 cm (38% ; 8/21). Even among tumors measuring ≤3 cm in diameter, cancer was seen at a frequency of 22% (7/32), indicating importance of careful follow-up by diagnostic imaging.

④Surgical pathologic findings in cases with main pancreatic-duct type IPMNs (Table 7)

There were a total of 11 cases of main pancreatic duct type carcinoma, the lesion being non-invasive in 5 cases, minimally invasive in 3 cases, and invasive in 3 cases, as shown in Table 7. A tall polypoid carcinoma in the main pancreatic duct was noted in 4 of the 5 cases of non-invasive carcinoma. In contrast, the protuberance in the main pancreatic duct wall was relatively low in height and broad-based in the cases of minimally invasive carcinoma and invasive carcinoma. There was no case of lymph node metastasis and the prognosis was favorable in the cases with non-invasive carcinoma as well as those with minimally invasive carcinoma.

⑤Surgical pathologic findings in case with mixed-type IPMNs (Table 8)

There were 12 cases of mixed-type carcinoma, i. e., 4 cases of non-invasive carcinoma, 1 case of minimally invasive carcinoma, and 7 cases of invasive carcinoma, as shown in Table 8. The carcinoma lesion was extensive, extending from the main pancreatic duct to the branch ducts in most cases, except Cases 3 and 6 shown in Table 8. Intraductal adenocarcinoma spread extensively, involving the main pancreatic duct and branch ducts of the entire pancreas in 3 cases (Cases 4, 8 and 11).

Table 7 Surgical pathologic findings in cases with main pancreatic-duct type IPMNs (Cancer Institute, 1979 to 2004)

Histologic type	Case	Age (yr.) Gender	Site	Size (mm)	n	Schematic illustration of resected specimen	Schematic illustration of cut section	Prognosis
Non-invasive	1	70 · Female	Head	34×20×23	(−)			Died of debility 12 years 10 months after diagnosis
	2	62 · Male	Head / Body	20×21×35 / 30×35×40	(−)			Died of debility 10 years 4 months after diagnosis
	3	65 · Female	Head	7×7×13	(−)			Surviving at 11 years 1 month after the diagnosis
	4	67 · Male	Body	37×28×8	(−)			Surviving at 8 years 6 months after diagnosis
	5	58 · Male	Head	80×25×25	(−)			Surviving at 3 years 6 months after diagnosis
Minimally invasive	6	57 · Female	Whole pancreas	55×180×40	(−)			Died of debility 16 years after diagnosis
	7	63 · Male	Body	25×18×25	(−)			Died 6 years 1 month after diagnosis Metachronous invasive carcinoma of the head of the pancreas
	8	56 · Male	Head	50×40×25	(−)			Died of cancer 5 years 11 months after diagnosis
Invasive	9	64 · Female	Body to tail	70×120×65	(+)			Died 9 months after diagnosis Myocardial infarction
	10	77 · Male	Whole pancreas	52×150×38	(+)			intravenous tumor thrombus Died of cancer 2 months after diagnosis
	11	60 · Female	Body to tail	40×25×17	(+)			Died of cancer 1 year after diagnosis

n: lymph node metastasis, MPD: Main pancreatic duct. CBD: Common bile duct, ∷, ■: Non-invasive carcinoma, ▨: Invasive carcinoma

⑥Surgical pathologic findings in case with branch-type IPMNs (Table 9)

Branch-type carcinoma, as shown in Table 9, was non-invasive in 8 cases, minimally invasive in 3 cases, and invasive in 4 cases (total 15 cases). Two groups of cases, one with tall intraductal elevation and the other with low intraductal elevation, were concurrently seen, irrespective of whether there was invasion. Non-invasive carcinoma cases and minimally invasive carcinoma cases accounted for 73% (11/15 cases); the prognosis was favorable in general, although 3 of 4 patients with invasive carcinoma died within a relatively short period.

3) Surgical therapeutic outcomes and surgical indications in IPMN

The postoperative survival curves of the 82 patients of IPMN treated by resection are presented in Table 10. The patients

Table 8 Surgical pathologic findings in cases with mixed-type IPMNs (Cancer Institute, 1979 to 2004)

Histologic type	Case	Age (yr.) Gender	Site	Size (mm)	n	Schematic illustration of resected specimen	Schematic illustration of cut section	Prognosis
Non-invasive	1	76・Female	Head to tail	70×40×35	(−)			Died of debility 3 years 3 months after diagnosis
	2*	55・Male	Head	35×50×17	(−)			Surviving at 18 years 4 month after the diagnosis
	3	64・Male	Head	25×22×22	(−)			Surviving at 8 years 3 month after the diagnosis
	4	72・Female	Whole pancreas	95×38×25	(−)			Surviving at 7 years after diagnosis
Minimally invasive	5	67・Male	Body to tail	60×40×20	(−)			Surviving at 9 years after diagnosis
Invasive	6	62・Female	Head	13×13×15	(−)			Died of cancer 3 years 5 months after diagnosis
	7	75・Male	Head	70×50×42	(+)			Died of Pneumonia 4 month after diagnosis
	8	67・Male	Whole pancreas	70×128×50	(+)			Died of cancer 2 years 4 months after diagnosis
	9	75・Female	Tail to body	106×55×40	(−)			Died of cancer 6 months after diagnosis
	10	47・Male	Body to tail	110×35×30	(−)			Surviving at 5 years 6 month after the diagnosis
	11	62・Female	Whole pancreas	220×100×80	(−)			Surviving at 4 years 8 month after the diagnosis
	12	69・Female	Head to tail	100×65×50	(−)			Surviving at 4 years 9 month after the diagnosis

n: lymph node metastasis, MPD: Main pancreatic duct, CBD: Common bile duct,
∷, ■: Non-invasive carcinoma, ▨: Invasive carcinoma
＊The final pathologic diagnosis in Case 2 was adenoma (high degree of atypia) in February 2013.

were grouped into the following 4 groups : benign (adenoma or hyperplasia), 44 cases ; non-invasive carcinoma, 17 cases ; minimally invasive carcinoma, 5 cases ; invasive carcinoma, 16 cases. The survival rates were determined with analysis for statistically significant intergroup differences using the log rank test (Table 10). Patients who died of other disorder postoperatively were censored as of the time of death and all cases of death were subjected to this assessment as such. There were significant differences in the prognosis between the benign group and the invasive carcinoma group ($p < 0.001$) and between the non-invasive carcinoma group and invasive carcinoma group ($p = 0.026$). The minimally

Table 9 Surgical pathologic findings in case with branch-type IPMNs (Cancer Institute, 1979 to 2004)

Histologic type	Case	Age (yr.) · Gender	Site	Size (mm)	n	Schematic illustration of resected specimen	Schematic illustration of cut section	Prognosis
Non-invasive	1	71 · Female	Body	50×20×7	(−)			Surviving at 9 years 10 month after the diagnosis
	2	58 · Female	Head	35×25×20	(−)			Surviving at 9 years 9 month after the diagnosis
	3	78 · Male	Head	33×31×20	(−)			Died of debility 5 months after diagnosis
	4	63 · Male	Head	20×5×32	(−)			Surviving at 15 years 9 month after diagnosis
	5	71 · Male	Head	40×23×12	(−)			Died of other disorder 1 years 2 months after diagnosis
	6	54 · Female	Head	25×24×10	(−)			Surviving at 4 years 9 month after diagnosis
	7	72 · Male	Body to head	35×25×12	(−)			Surviving at 4 years 8 month after diagnosis
	8	75 · Male	Body	18×13×6	(−)			Surviving at 3 years 6 month after diagnosis
Minimally invasive	9	64 · Male	Head	35×30×30	(−)			Died of other disorder 8 years 3 months after diagnosis
	10	65 · Male	Head	33×31×20	(−)			Died of debility 8 years 2 months after diagnosis
	11	63 · Male	Head	30×28×15	(−)			Surviving at 6 years 8 month after diagnosis
Invasive	12	73 · Male	Head	38×30×38	(+)			Died of cancer 7 months after diagnosis
	13	72 · Male	Head	25×25×23	(−)			Died of cancer 3 years 3 months after diagnosis
	14	65 · Female	Head	35×35×25	(−)			Died of cancer 9 months after diagnosis
	15	72 · Female	Head to body	25×20×14	(−)			Surviving at 3 years 7 month after diagnosis

n: lymph node metastasis, MPD: Main pancreatic duct. CBD: Common bile duct,
∷, ■: Non-invasive carcinoma, ▨: Invasive carcinoma
*The final pathologic diagnosis in Case 10 was invasive carcinoma rather than minimally invasive carcinoma in February 2013.

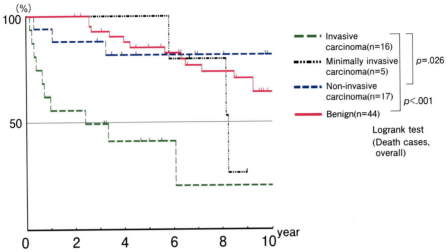

Table 10 Survival curves by the histologic type of IPMN

Table 11 Survival rate by the histologic type of IPMN

	5年	10年	50%	
Invasive	41.0%	21.0%	29月	*, **
Minimally invasive	100.0%		99月	
Non-invasive	81.9%	81.9%	153月	**
Benign	85.3%	60.1%	198月	*

invasive carcinoma group, of which there were relatively few cases (5 cases), exhibited a survival curve essentially comparable to that for the non-invasive carcinoma group until 8 years post-operation. The invasive carcinoma group showed the poorest prognosis among the 4 groups, with 5- and 10-year survival rates of 41% and 21%, respectively; nonetheless, the prognosis of this group was still better than that of the cases with the usual type of invasive carcinoma of the pancreas (Table 11).

The following were inferred from the above-described surgical pathological assessments of the 82 cases of IPMN treated by resection:

①The frequencies of cancer in intraductal pancreatic tumors classified by the tumor location were as follows: 91.7% in main pancreatic-duct type tumors, 70.6% in mixed-type tumors, and 28.3% in branch-type tumors. Thus, the frequencies of malignancy were higher in the main pancreatic duct-type and mixed-type tumors.

②When classified by the tumor size, the frequency of cancer in the 53 cases of branch-type IPMN was relatively high in tumors of large diameter: 50% (8/16) in cases with lesions measuring 3.0-4.0 cm in diameter and 38% (8/21) in cases with lesions measuring >3 cm in diameter.

③The prognosis of minimally invasive carcinoma confined to within the pancreas, with no evidence of lymphogenous or hematogenous metastasis, was as favorable as that of non-invasive carcinoma; therefore, this type of tumor should be carefully differentiated by histopathology from invasive carcinoma derived from other types of intraductal papillary tumors of the pancreas.

Based on the above outcomes of surgical treatment, we propose the following surgical indications in cases of IPMN:

(1) Lesions of the main pancreatic-duct type or mixed type

(2) Lesions of the branch type exceeding 3 cm in diameter, unless any mural nodule is suspected in the dilated pancreatic duct on diagnostic imaging

(3) Lesions of the branch type, irrespective of the size, that show a rapid increase of the tumor size or increase of mural nodules, or in which invasion of adjacent structures is suspected on follow-up diagnostic imaging.

References

1) Ohashi K, Murakami Y, Maruyama M, et al. Four cases of mucin-producing cancer of the pancreas : Focusing on specific findings of the papilla of vater. Progress of Digestive Endoscopy **20** : 348-351, 1982.
2) Japan Pancreas Society (eds). General Rules for the Study of Pancreatic Cancer (The 5th Edition). Kanehara & Co, LTD. 2002.
3) Longnecker DS, Hruban RH, Adler G, et al. Intraductal papillary-mucinous neoplasms of the pancreas. In : Hamilton SR, Aaltonen LA (eds) World Health Organization Classification of Tumours. Pathology and Genetics of Tumours of the Digestive System. Lyon : IARC Press, 237-240, 2000.
4) Ohashi K, Tajiri H, Gondo M, et al. A case of resection of cystic adenocarcinoma of the pancreas forming a biliopancreatic fistula. Progress of Digestive Endoscopy **17** : 261-264 : 1980.
5) Murakami Y, Gondo M, Ohashi K, et al. A case of multifocal papillary ductal carcinoma in situ in the pancreatic head and body. Progress of Digestive Endoscopy **19** : 304-307 : 1981.
6) Murakami Y, Ohashi K, Takekoshi T, et al. Pre- and post-operative ERCP findings of mucin-producing cancer of the pancreas. Progress of Digestive Endoscopy **23** : 338-341 : 1983.
7) Ohashi K. The history of so-called mucin-producing cancer of the pancreas over 15 years by the researcher who first described this entity. Journal of Biliary Tract & Pancreas **18** : 609-613, 1997.
8) Takagi K, Ikeda S, Nakagawa Y, et al. Retrograde pancreatography and cholangiography by fiber duodenoscope. Gastroenterology **59** : 445-452, 1970.
9) Takagi K, Takahashi T, Hori M, et al. Small carcinoma of head of the pancreas discovered by the clue of transitory elevation of urinary amylase level. Stomach and Intestine **15** : 637-640, 1980.
10) Takagi K. Early Diagnosis of pancreatic carcinoma. Asian Med J **33** : 385-393, 1990.

Case 1 Relatively typical main-pancreatic duct type intraductal papillary-mucinous carcinoma (IPMC) without pancreatic duct invasion that required distinction from the mixed-type

Case: A man in his 60s
Chief complaint: Asymptomatic (lesion discovered by ultrasonography [US])
Family history: Lung cancer in one uncle, prostate cancer in another
Past history: Left cataract surgery at age 43, oral antihypertensive drug treatment for hypertension since age 54
Smoking and drinking history: Drinking, drank one can of beer/day for 35 years ; smoking, smoked 20 cigarettes/day for 40 years
Present illness: In February 1999, dilatation of the main pancreatic duct was detected by abdominal US during a health checkup at a local facility. The patient was admitted to the same facility for detailed examination. Tests led to a diagnosis of mucus-producing tumor of the tail of the pancreas.
  In late April, he was referred to our Department of Surgery for surgery. The patient requested that the surgery be performed in January of the following year for job-related reasons.
Abdominal US (Fig. 1): An intramural nodule was detected in the dilated main pancreatic duct lumen in the pancreatic tail.
Endoscopic US (Fig. 2): An intramural nodule protruding into the lumen was visible in the dilated pancreatic duct in the pancreatic tail.
Contrast-enhanced computed tomography (CT) (Fig. 3): The main pancreatic duct in the pancreatic tail was dilated, and the presence of an intramural nodule was suggested.
Magnetic resonance cholangiopancreatography (MRCP) (Fig. 4): The main pancreatic duct in the pancreatic tail region showed cystiform dilatation, accompanied by dilatation of some of the adjoining pancreatic duct branches.
Endoscopic findings of the duodenal papilla (Fig. 5), **endoscopic retrograde cholangiopancreatography (ERCP)** (Fig. 6): The opening of the major papilla was slightly dilated. The main pancreatic duct in the pancreatic tail region showed cystiform dilatation, with radiolucencies seen sporadically within the lumen.
Angiography findings (Fig. 7): A sign of small artery compression in the pancreatic tail was visible.
Surgical procedure (Fig. 8): In mid-January 2000, distal pancreatectomy was performed (operation time, 3 hours 35 minutes ; blood loss, 315 g).
Macroscopic observation of the resected specimen (Fig. 9): On the anterior plane of the pancreatic tail, a part of the cystic lesion was visible.
Findings on pancreatography of the resected specimen (Fig. 10): Cystiform dilatation of the main pancreatic duct was visible in the pancreatic tail region.
Postoperative course: The patient survived for 8 years 6 months after the surgery.

Blood Cell Counts	
WBC	6,100 /μL
RBC	4.51×10^6 /μL
Hb	13.8 g/dL
Ht	42.1 %
Plt	214×10^3 /μL

Tumor Markers	
CEA	1.1 ng/mL
CA19-9	7.0 U/mL
DUPAN-2	<25 U/mL
Elastase 1	230 ng/dL

Biochemistry	
TP	6.6 g/dL
Alb	3.7 g/dL
T-Bil	0.6 mg/dL
γ-GTP	34 U/L
ALP	248 U/L
GOT	26 U/L
GPT	18 U/L
Amy	138 U/L
Glu	87 mg/dL
BUN	15 mg/dL
Crea	0.98 mg/dL

I. Imaging Findings

Fig. 1 Abdominal US (1)

Abdominal US (2)

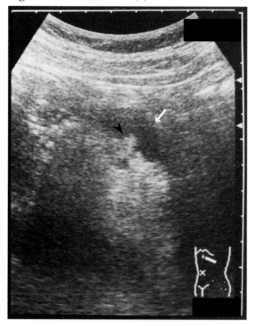
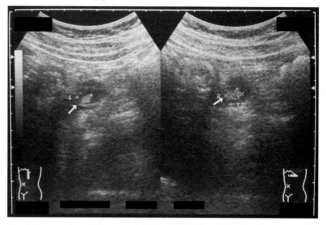

An intramural nodule was visible within the dilated main pancreatic duct lumen in the pancreatic tail (→).

Dilatation of the main pancreatic duct was seen in the body/tail region (→), with findings suggestive of the presence of an intramural nodule protruding into the pancreatic duct lumen (▶).

Fig. 2 Endoscopic US

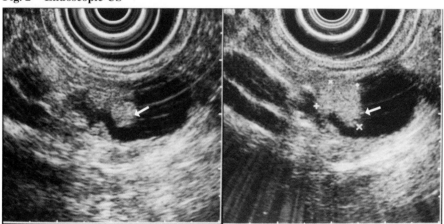

An intramural nodule protruding into the lumen was visible in the dilated main pancreatic duct in the pancreatic tail (→).

Fig. 3 Contrast-enhanced CT

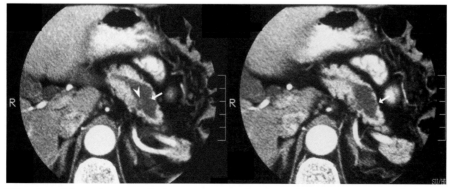

Dilatation of the main pancreatic duct was seen in the pancreatic body to tail region (→), with suspected presence of an intramural nodule (▶).

Fig. 4 MRCP

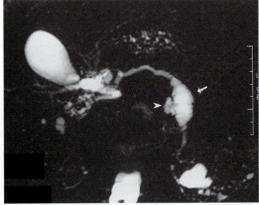

Cystiform dilatation of the main pancreatic duct was seen in the pancreatic body to tail region (→), accompanied by dilatation of some of the adjoining pancreatic duct branches (▶).

Fig. 5 Endoscopic findings of the duodenal papilla

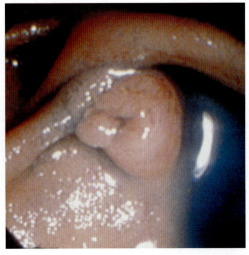

The opening of the major papilla was slightly enlarged.

Fig. 6 ERCP (1)

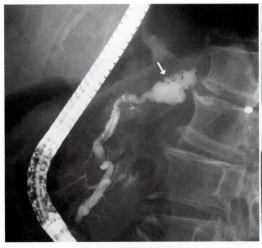

Cystiform dilatation of the main pancreatic duct seen in the pancreatic body to tail region (→).

ERCP (2)

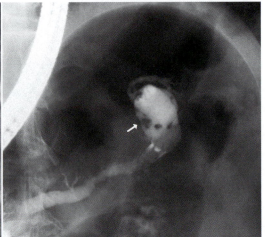

When the part of the main pancreatic duct showing cystiform dilatation was compressed, radiolucencies were noted sporadically within the lumen (→).

Fig. 7 Angiography

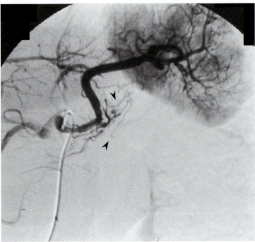

Evidence of slight sign of compression was visible in the small arteries of the pancreatic tail (▶), however, there was no sign of encasement.

II. Surgical Findings

Fig. 8　Surgical findings

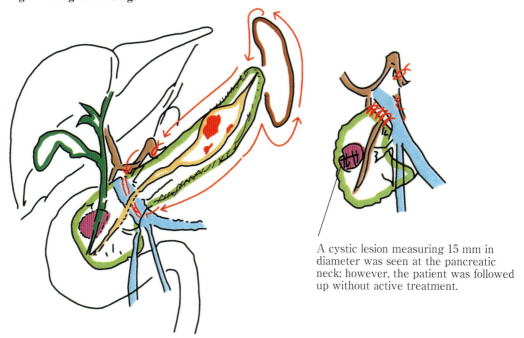

A cystic lesion measuring 15 mm in diameter was seen at the pancreatic neck; however, the patient was followed up without active treatment.

Fig. 9　Resected specimen (anterior view)

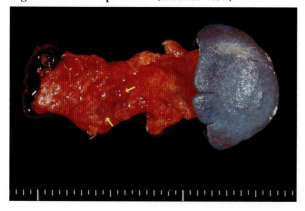

The cystic lesion was partially visible on the anterior plane of the pancreatic tail (→).

Fig. 10　Pancreatography of the resected specimen

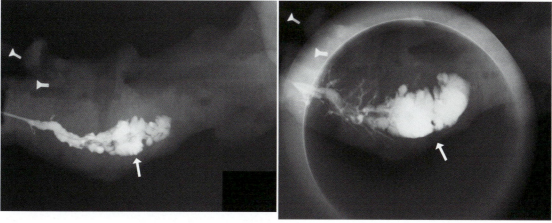

A part of the main pancreatic duct showing cystiform dilatation was visible in the pancreatic tail region (→).

III. Pathological Findings

Fig. 11　Tissue architecture of the resected specimen

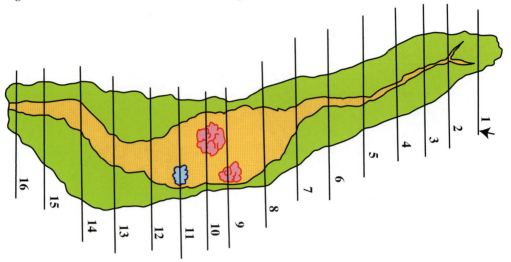

Red part：cancer, Blue part：adenoma

Fig. 12　Findings of the cut surfaces of the resected specimen

1. Findings of the cut surfaces of all the sections of the resected specimen

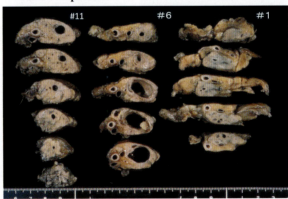

2. Photograph of the cut surface of section #9

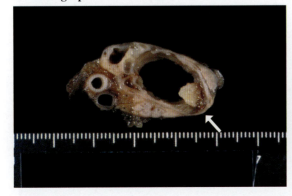

3. Photograph of the cut surface of section #10 reversed

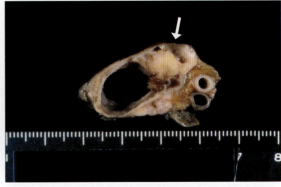

Case 1 Relatively typical main-pancreatic duct type intraductal papillary-mucinous carcinoma (IPMC) without pancreatic duct invasion that required distinction from the mixed-type 21

Fig. 13 Findings of the cut surfaces of all the sections of the resected specimen

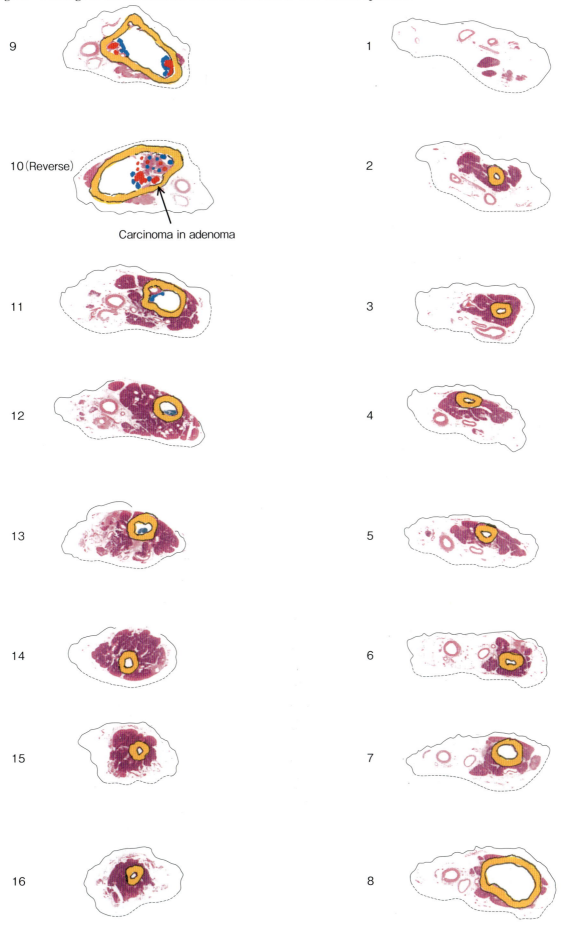

Red part : cancer, Blue part : adenoma

Fig. 14 Collation of the pre- and postoperative endoscopic retrograde pancreatography (ERP) images with projection views of the resected specimen

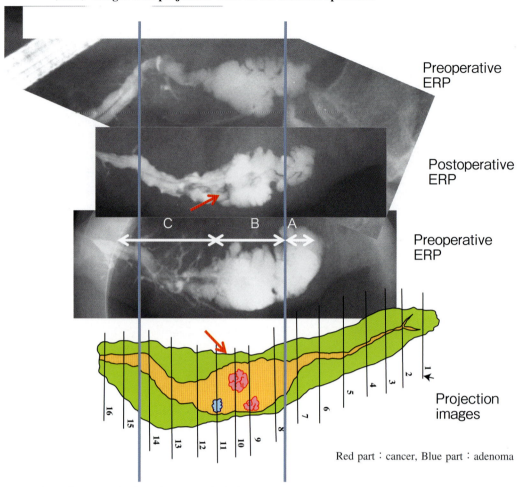

Area A : The main pancreatic duct showed marked dilatation cranial to section #7. Area B : The radiolucent region revealed by ERP after surgery for the main lesion (papillary proliferative lesion) indicated by the red arrow corresponded to the papillary lesion inside the main pancreatic duct. Area C : Slightly dilated region of the main pancreatic duct

Area A #7 and 8

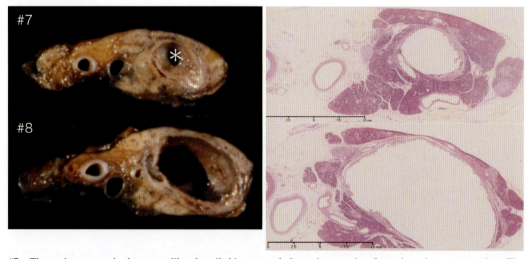

#7. The main pancreatic duct was dilated until this part and showed narrowing from the subsequent section. The dilated main pancreatic duct was visible on the cut plane of the photographed section, with the deeper plane showing narrowing of the main pancreatic duct (＊).

#8. The dilated main pancreatic duct was clearly visible. On more detailed observation, the wall was found to show a short papillary lesion. This papillary lesion was mild in terms of the severity of the atypia and appeared to be spreading uninterruptedly within the pancreatic duct.

Area B #9

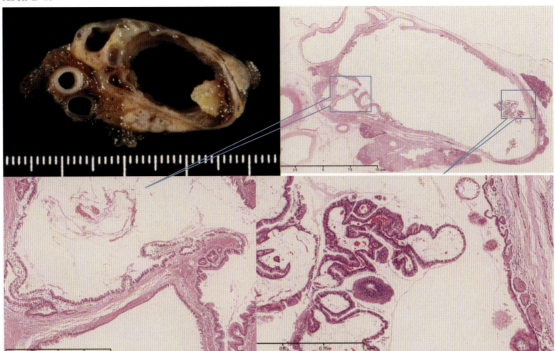

a, b, c, d. The wall inside the dilated main pancreatic duct and the pancreatic duct branch showed short papillary lesions. The cellular atypia was mild, which led to the diagnosis of adenoma. d. A photomicrograph of the section showing a slightly tall papillary proliferative lesion (×5 mm) in a part of the main pancreatic duct wall.

A diagnosis of moderately atypical adenoma was made. This lesion corresponded to the radiolucent area visible in the ERP images.

#10 Reversed

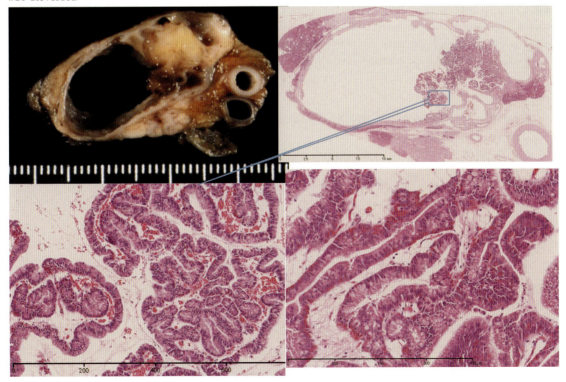

a, b, c. A tall papillary proliferative lesion was visible on the inner wall of the main pancreatic duct extending to a pancreatic duct branch. This lesion corresponded to the arrow in the ERP image (Fig. 14). c. Histologically, the lesion comprised an adenoma for the most part, however, foci of cancer with marked structural and cellular atypia were noted (d).

Collation of the preoperative images with the histological picture

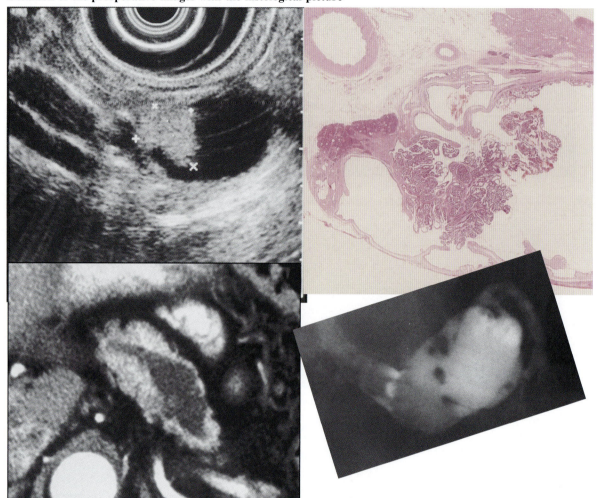

The intramural nodule revealed by endoscopic US appeared to correspond to the papillary proliferative lesion in the wall of the dilated main pancreatic duct and pancreatic duct branch noted on the reverse plane of #10. The papillary proliferative lesion was visible as a radiolucent area on the contrast-enhanced CT and compressed ERP images.

Histopathologic diagnosis

Intraductal papillary-mucinous neoplasm (IPMN), carcinoma in adenoma, non-invasive, of the body of the pancreas MPD type, 37 × 28 × 8 mm, N0 (0/9)

Pathologist's comment : The major lesion was located in the dilated main pancreatic duct, partially spreading into a pancreatic duct branch. Two elevated lesions were seen. Histologically, mostly mild atypia was seen, based on which adenoma was diagnosed. In some foci, however, severe atypia was observed, which led to the diagnosis of IPMN, "Cancer in adenoma."

Clinician's comment : This was the case of a patient who underwent detailed examination and surgery after US during a health checkup revealed cystiform dilatation of the main pancreatic duct in the pancreatic tail. Identification of the intraductal papillary tumor was difficult by US and CT, however, the tumor was clearly visualized by endoscopic US. When the sections were observed macroscopically, the lesion appeared to spread from the main pancreatic duct to a primary branch of the main duct, however, the main lesion was located in the main pancreatic duct, which led to the judgment of the tumor being of the main pancreatic-duct type. Distinction between the main-pancreatic duct type and mixed-type sometimes proves difficult, as in this case. MRCP revealed a cystic lesion measuring 15 mm in diameter in the pancreatic neck, and the patient is currently under close follow-up. The lesion has grown to 20 mm, however, its features remain unchanged.

Case 2 Invasive cancer of pancreatic tail intraductal papillary-mucinous neoplasm (IPMN) origin presenting with typical signs of mucinous carcinoma

Case: A woman in her 60s
Chief complaint: Pain of the epigastric region radiating to the left back
Family history: Gastric cancer in grandfather and father, liver cancer in an elder brother
Past history: Conservative therapy for gastric ulcer at our hospital since age 50, diabetes since age 59
Smoking and drinking history: Drinking (−); smoking (−)
Present illness: In mid-August 2001, she consulted our Department of Internal Medicine for pain in the epigastric region radiating to the left back. Abdominal computed tomography (CT) revealed dilatation of the main pancreatic duct in the pancreatic tail, and the patient was admitted for more detailed examination.
Abdominal ultrasonography (US) (Fig. 1): Dilatation of the main pancreatic duct and a hypoechoic mass were noted in the pancreatic tail. Poorly demarcated hypoechoic areas were seen around the main pancreatic duct in the pancreatic body.
Transgastric endoscopic ultrasonography (Fig. 2): A hypoechoic mass, about 4 cm in size, was visible in the pancreatic tail. The hypoechoic area was contiguous with the pancreatic body.
Abdominal CT (Fig. 3): The main pancreatic duct in the pancreatic tail was dilated; adjacent to the dilated pancreatic duct was a low-density mass, which was contiguous with the pancreatic body.
Findings as to the papilla (Fig. 4): The opening of the major papilla was slightly enlarged.
Findings on endoscopic retrograde cholangiopancreatography (ERCP) (Fig. 5): The cystiform dilatation of the main pancreatic duct was visible in the pancreatic tail, with shadow defects visible in the lumen. The main pancreatic duct towards the pancreatic body showed irregular stenotic lesions.
Angiography findings (Fig. 6): Dim tumor staining was visible in the pancreatic tail.
Surgical procedure (Fig. 7): In late September, pancreatic body and tail resection was performed (operation time, 7 hours 5 minutes; blood loss, 525 g).
Macroscopic observation of the resected specimen (Fig. 8): The anterior plane of the pancreatic tail contained a grayish-white area, suggesting exposure of the tumor.
Findings on pancreatography of the resected specimen (Fig. 9): A partially dilated pancreatic duct was visualized in the pancreatic tail, accompanied by shadow defects inside the lumen, along with several pancreatic ducts with irregular lumina towards the tail region.
Postoperative course: The patient died from cancer at one year.

Blood Cell Counts	
WBC	9,000 /µL
RBC	4.39×10^6 /µL
Hb	14.5 g/dL
Ht	42.8 %
Plt	321×10^3 /µL

Tumor Markers	
CEA	0.8 ng/mL
CA19-9	80.6 U/mL

Biochemistry	
TP	7.8 g/dL
Alb	4.7 g/dL
T-Bil	0.6 mg/dL
D-Bil	0.2 mg/dL
γ-GTP	26 U/L
ALP	264 U/L
GOT	19 U/L
GPT	26 U/L
Amy	634 U/L
P-Amy	500 U/L
Glu	160 mg/dL
BUN	15 mg/dL
Crea	0.98 mg/dL

I. Imaging Findings

Fig. 1 Abdominal US

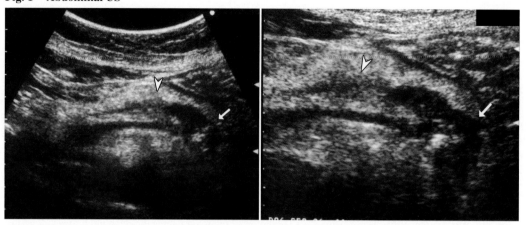

Dilatation of the main pancreatic duct and a hypoechoic mass were noted in the pancreatic tail (→). Poorly demarcated hypoechoic areas were seen around the main pancreatic duct in the pancreatic body (►).

Fig. 2 Transgastric endoscopic US

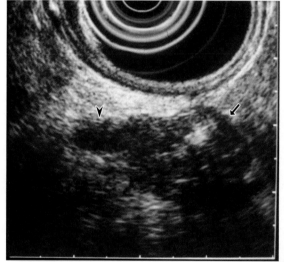

A quasi-circular hypoechoic mass, about 4 cm in size, was visible in the pancreatic tail (→), and the hypoechoic mass was contiguous with the pancreatic body (►).

Fig. 3 Abdominal CT

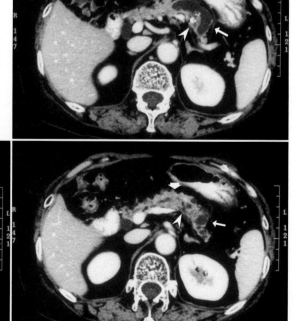

The main pancreatic duct in the pancreatic tail was dilated (→); adjacent to it was a low-density mass with an inhomogeneous internal density (►) that was contiguous with the pancreatic body (◆).

Fig. 4 Duodenal papilla endoscopy

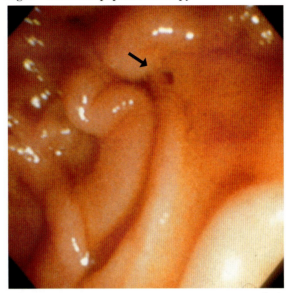

The opening of the major papilla was slightly enlarged (→).

Fig. 5 ERCP

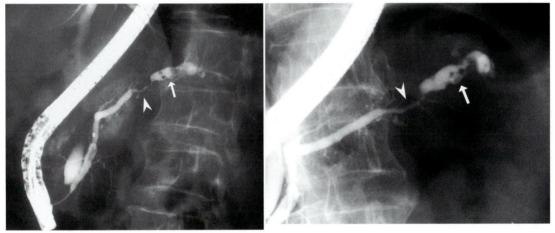

Cystiform dilatation of a part of the main pancreatic duct in the pancreatic tail was seen, with shadow defects inside the lumen (→). The segment of the main pancreatic duct close to the pancreatic body showed irregular stenosis (▶).

Fig. 6 Angiography

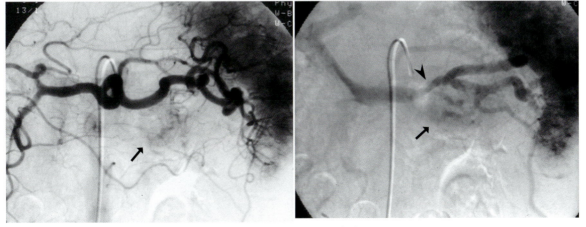

A circular area with dim tumor staining was visible in the pancreatic tail (→), accompanied by encasement of small artery and vein. The splenic vein showed stenosis (▶).

II. Surgical Findings

Fig. 7 Surgical findings

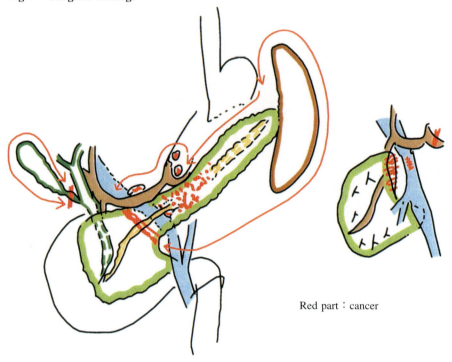

Red part : cancer

Fig. 8 Resected specimen (anterior view)

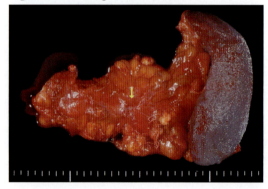

A grayish-white area showing some shrinkage, suggestive of exposed tumor, was visible in the anterior plane of the pancreatic tail region (→).

Fig. 9 Pancreatography of the resected specimen

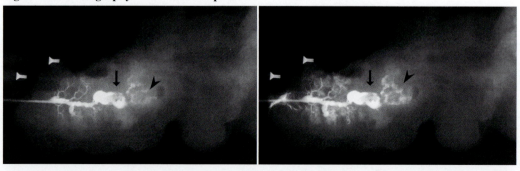

Injection of contrast material into the stump of the main pancreatic duct led to visualization of the dilated part of the duct in the pancreatic tail, with shadow defects visualized within the lumen (→). The main pancreatic duct segment towards the pancreatic body was irregular ; in addition, several pancreatic duct branches with irregular lumina were visualized within the tail region (►).

III. Pathological Findings

Fig. 10 Tissue architecture of the resected specimen

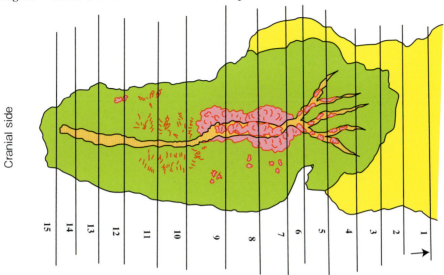

Red part : cancer

Fig. 11 Findings of the cut surfaces of the resected specimen

1. Photograph of the cut surfaces of all the sections of the resected specimen

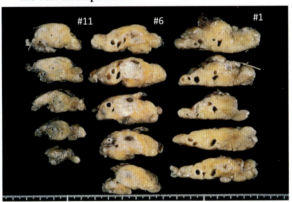

2. Photograph of the cut surfaces of sections #6 to 11

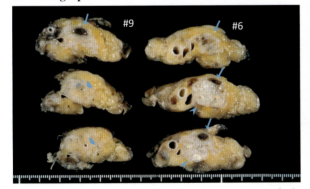

The main pancreatic duct was dilated in the pancreatic tail (→), with a muconodular cancer seen on the dorsal side (►). The main pancreatic duct segment towards the pancreatic body was narrowed (⇾), surrounded by grayish-white invasive cancer.

3. Photograph of the cut surfaces of sections #7 to 8

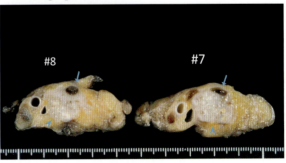

The main pancreatic duct was dilated in the pancreatic tail region (→), and a grayish-white mucinous node with yellow-white internal calcification was seen on the dorsal side (►).

Fig. 12 Findings of the cut surfaces of all sections of the resected specimen

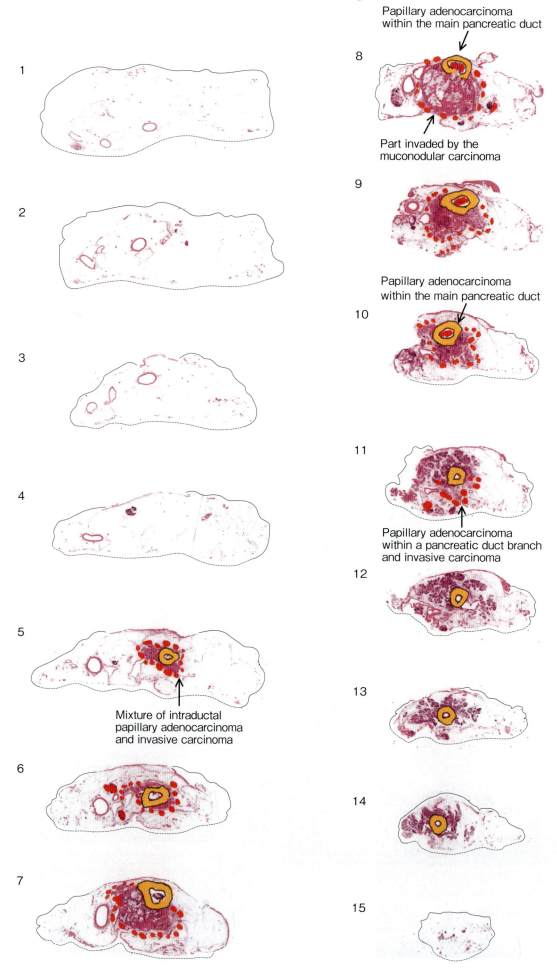

Fig. 13 Collation of the pre- and postoperative endoscopic retrograde pancreatography (ERP) images with the postoperative projection views of the resected specimen

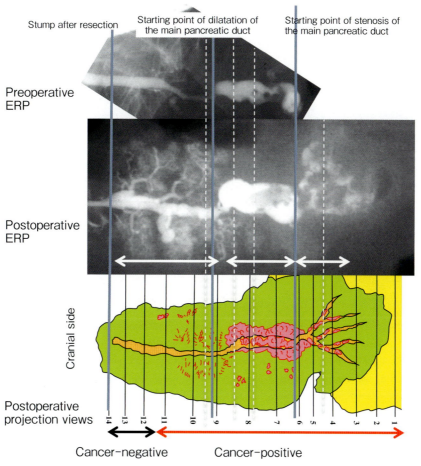

Areas until section #12 from the cranial side were negative for cancer and areas caudal to section #11 were positive. The extent of cancer spread and invasion varied among the areas cranial to the dilated part of the main pancreatic duct, the dilated part of the duct, and the area caudal to the dilated part. Area A, caudal area showing an irregularly branching pancreatic duct ; Area B, dilated part of the main pancreatic duct ; Area C, cranial area showing slight dilatation of the main pancreatic duct

Area A #5

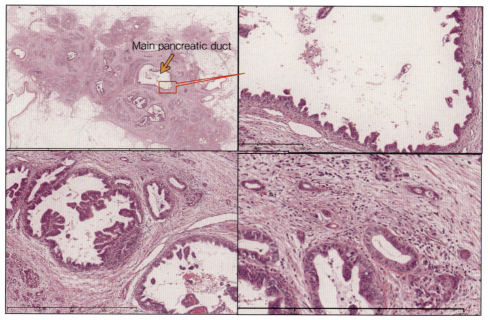

a. A slightly dilated main pancreatic duct and atrophic pancreatic parenchyma were visible. b. A cancerous tumor in the form of a short papillary growth was seen in the main pancreatic duct. c. The pancreatic duct branches were slightly dilated, with cancer spreading on the wall. d. Diffusely invading small foci of cancer were visible in the surrounding region.

Area B #8

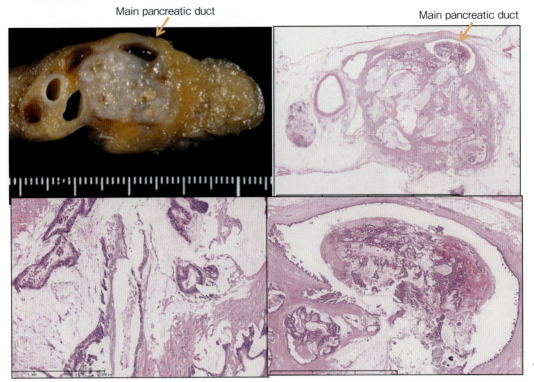

a. Photograph of a section. The dilated main pancreatic duct and the mucinous node within the pancreatic parenchyma were visible. b. A tumor plug-like proliferative lesion was noted within the main pancreatic duct. c. Area of the pancreatic parenchyma invaded by the cancer. Mucinous nodes were visible, which led to the diagnosis of mucinous carcinoma. d. Histological findings at the origin of the embolus-like proliferative lesion. The invasive mucinous carcinoma was contiguous with the main pancreatic duct at this point (flow of mucus from the main pancreatic duct into the stroma was visible).

Area C, slice #9 First specimen of the main pancreatic duct showing transition from stenosis to dilatation

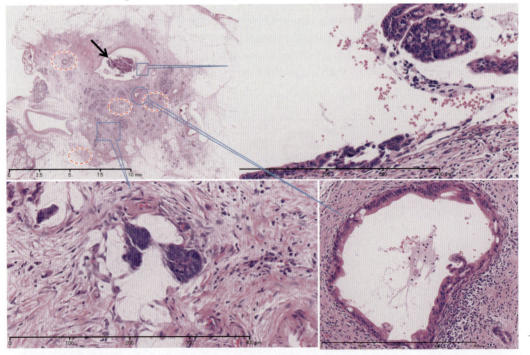

a. Cancerous papillary growth visible within the main pancreatic duct (→). Cancer growing in the form of an embolus within the main pancreatic duct, with the pancreatic parenchyma around this area being relatively well-preserved. Cancer was visible within the region denoted with a circled in red broken line (branching pancreatic duct showing cancer spread) and the region denoted by the square (invasive carcinoma). b. Cancer spreading on the main pancreatic duct wall. c. Invasive carcinoma. d. Cancer spreading within the wall of a pancreatic duct branch

Collation of the preoperative images with the histologic features

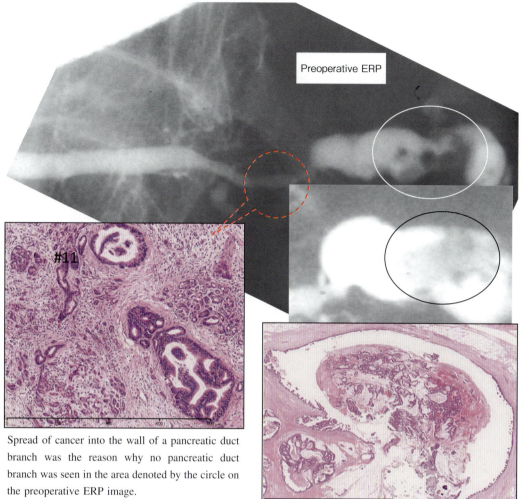

Spread of cancer into the wall of a pancreatic duct branch was the reason why no pancreatic duct branch was seen in the area denoted by the circle on the preoperative ERP image.

The shadow defects within the main pancreatic duct seen on the pre- and postoperative ERP images were attributable to the embolus-like growth of the cancer within the main pancreatic duct.

Histopathologic diagnosis

Intraductal papillary-mucinous carcinoma, invasive, of the tail of the pancreas

MPD type, 40×25×17 mm, INF b, ly3, v0, ne1, s0, rpe, pw (−), ew (+), N2 (7/17, 7), 8), 9), 14))

Pathologist's comment: Histological distinction between mucinous carcinoma and invasive carcinoma of IPMN origin was difficult in this case. A diagnosis of invasive carcinoma of IPMN origin was made on the basis of the cystiform dilatation of the main pancreatic duct filled with mucus, the manner of spread of the intraepithelial components within the main pancreatic duct, and the presence of the papillary proliferative lesion. In this case, the relationship of the papillary proliferative lesion of the main pancreatic duct to the mucinous carcinoma was controversial, although continuity (formation of muconodular cancer through invasion of the IPMN beyond the wall) was confirmed. The histological appearance of the transition was very clearly depicted.

Clinician's comment: During preoperative diagnostic imaging, the relationship between the circular mass in the pancreatic tail showing calcification and the mass in the adjacent pancreatic body around the stenosed main pancreatic duct was not clear. However, histopathological examination led to the diagnosis of invasion of the area surrounding the main pancreatic duct in the pancreatic body region by the invasive carcinoma arising in the pancreatic tail. This was a valuable case where both the findings of diagnostic imaging and the pathological findings were quite noteworthy.

Case 3 Mixed-type non-invasive intraductal papillary-mucinous carcinoma (IPMC) of the pancreatic body spreading widely within a secondary branch of the pancreatic duct

Case: A woman in her 70s
Chief complaint: Asymptomatic (lesion discovered by abdominal ultrasonography [US])
Family history: Gastric cancer in mother, colorectal cancer in aunt
Past history: Appendectomy at age 17
Smoking and drinking history: Drinking (−); smoking (−)
Present illness: In November 1997, the patient visited a local facility to undergo an abdominal US, and the abdominal US revealed main pancreatic duct dilatation.
In early January 1998, she was referred to our hospital.
Abdominal US (Fig. 1): Dilatation was noted in a branch of the pancreatic duct in the pancreatic body.
Endoscopic US (Fig. 2): The main pancreatic duct and adjacent pancreatic duct branches in the pancreatic body were dilated, with small lesions suggestive of intramural nodules seen sporadically within the lumen.
Magnetic resonance cholangiopancreatography (MRCP) (Fig. 3): A cystic lesion composed of overlapping dilated pancreatic duct branches was visualized in the pancreatic body.
Contrast-enhanced abdominal computed tomography (CT) (Fig. 4): A dilated main pancreatic duct and pancreatic duct branches were seen in the pancreatic body.
Findings on endoscopic retrograde cholangiopancreatography (ERCP) and endoscopy of the duodenal papilla (Fig. 5): The opening of the major papilla was dilated, with mucus discharge.
ERCP findings (Fig. 6): The main pancreatic duct was dilated from the pancreatic head to the pancreatic tail, accompanied by dilatation of the pancreatic duct branches in the pancreatic body.
Surgical procedure (Fig. 7): In mid-May, caudal pancreatectomy (subtotal) and intraoperative pancreatoscopy were carried out (operation time, 6 hours 40 minutes; blood loss, 195 g).
Findings on intraoperative pancreatoscopy (Fig. 8): A milky-white elevated lesion and redness were noted within the main pancreatic duct in the pancreatic body.
Findings of the anterior plane of the resected specimen (Fig. 9): No evident exposure of the tumor or the cystic lesion
Pancreatography of the resected specimen (Fig. 10): Dilatation of the pancreatic duct branches was visible in the pancreatic body, but there was no evident radiolucency.
Postoperative course: The patient survived for 9 years 10 months after the surgery.

Blood Cell Counts	
WBC	4,000 /μL
RBC	4.68×10^6 /μL
Hb	13.0 g/dL
Ht	40.1 %
Plt	168×10^3 /μL

Tumor Markers	
CEA	1.3 ng/mL
CA19-9	2.5 U/mL
DUPAN-2	<25 U/mL
Elastase 1	180 ng/dL

Biochemistry	
TP	7.5 g/dL
Alb	4.4 g/dL
T-Bil	0.6 mg/dL
γ-GTP	20 U/L
ALP	300 U/L
GOT	18 U/L
GPT	10 U/L
T-chol	259 mg/dL
Amy	119 U/L
Glu	103 mg/dL
BUN	10 mg/dL
Crea	0.6 mg/dL

I. Imaging Findings

Fig. 1 Abdominal US (transverse scanning of the pancreatic body)

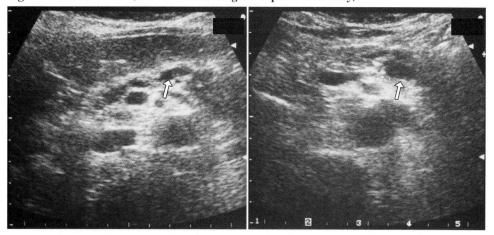

Dilatation of a branch of the pancreatic duct was visible in the pancreatic body (→).

Fig. 2 Endoscopic US (transgastric scanning)

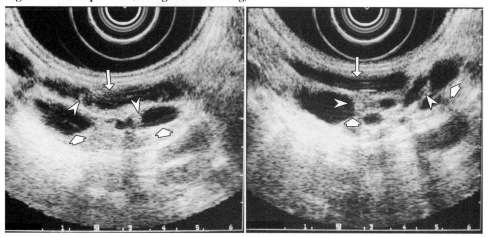

The main pancreatic duct and adjacent pancreatic duct branches (⇨) in the pancreatic body were dilated (→), with small lesions appearing like intramural nodules seen sporadically within the lumen (▶).

Fig. 3 MRCP

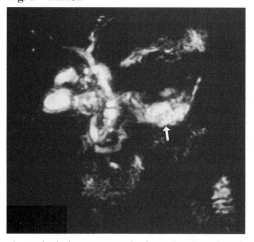

A cystic lesion composed of overlapping dilated pancreatic duct branches was visualized in the pancreatic body (→).

Fig. 4 Contrast-enhanced CT（Slice # assigned, beginning with the most cranial one）

1. #2   2. #5

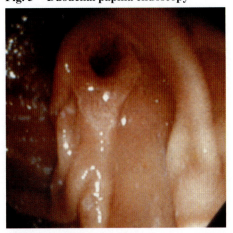

A dilated main pancreatic duct（→）and pancreatic duct branches（➤）were seen in the pancreatic body. The dilatation of the pancreatic duct extends to the pancreatic tail（⬇）.

Fig. 5 Duodenal papilla endoscopy

The opening of the major papilla was enlarged, with mucus discharge.

Fig. 6 ERCP（1）

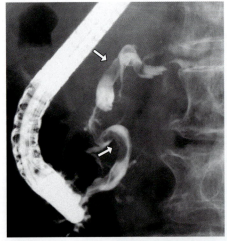

Dilatation was seen in the main pancreatic duct and pancreatic duct branches in the head and body of the pancreas, with radioluencies seen in the dilated ducts, possibly reflecting mucus retention（→）.

Endoscopic retrograde pancreatography（ERP）（2）

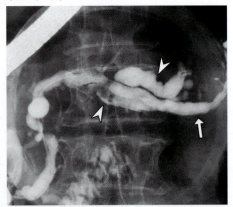

The main pancreatic duct was dilated from the pancreatic head to the pancreatic tail（→）, accompanied by dilatation of the pancreatic duct branches in the pancreatic body（➤）.

II. Surgical Findings

Fig. 7 Surgical findings

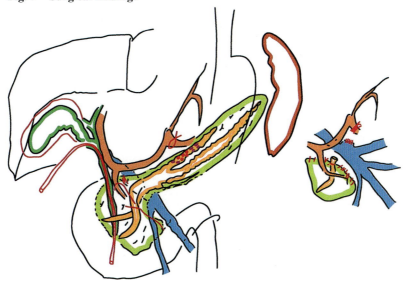

Fig. 8 Intraoperative pancreatoscopy

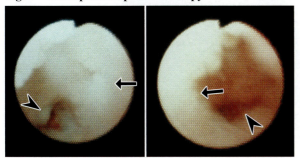

Within the main pancreatic duct in the pancreatic body region, a milky-white elevated lesion (→) and redness (▶) were visible.

Fig. 9 Resected specimen (anterior view)

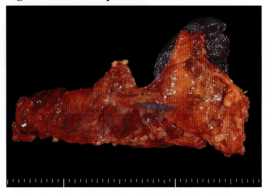

There was no evident exposure of the tumor or the cystic lesion.

Fig. 10 Pancreatography of the resected specimen

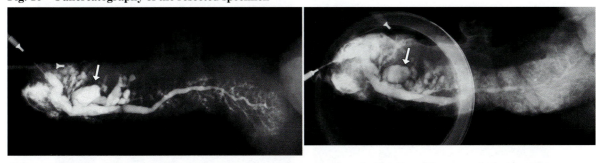

Following injection of the contrast material from the stump at the pancreatic neck, dilatation of the pancreatic duct branches was seen in the pancreatic body region (→), but there was no evident radiolucency.

III. Pathological Findings

Fig. 11 Tissue architecture of the resected specimen

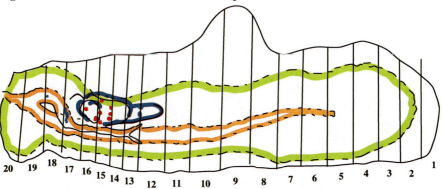

Red part : cancer, Blue part : adenoma

Fig. 12 Findings of the cut surfaces of the resected specimen
1. Photograph of the cut surfaces of all the sections of the resected specimen

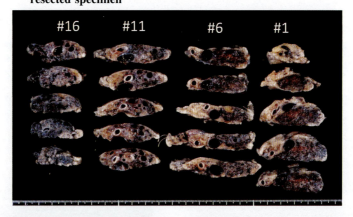

2. Photograph of the cut surface of section #13

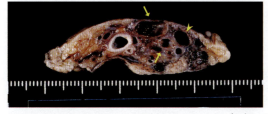

In contact with the dilated main pancreatic duct (➤), a group of dilated pancreatic duct branches was also visible (→).

3. Photograph of the cut surface of section #14

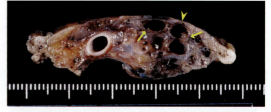

Within the dilated main pancreatic duct (➤) and dilated pancreatic duct branches, there were small papillary elevations (→).

4. Photograph of the cut surface of section #15

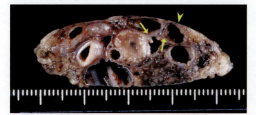

Within the dilated main pancreatic duct (➤) and the dilated pancreatic duct branches, there were small papillary elevations (→).

5. Photograph of the cut surface of section #16

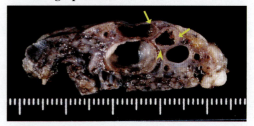

Within the dilated main pancreatic duct (➤) and the dilated branching pancreatic ducts, there were minimal papillary elevations (→).

Case 3 Mixed-type non-invasive intraductal papillary-mucinous carcinoma (IPMC) of the pancreatic body spreading widely within a secondary branch of the pancreatic duct 39

Fig. 13 Findings of the cut surfaces of all the sections of the resected specimen

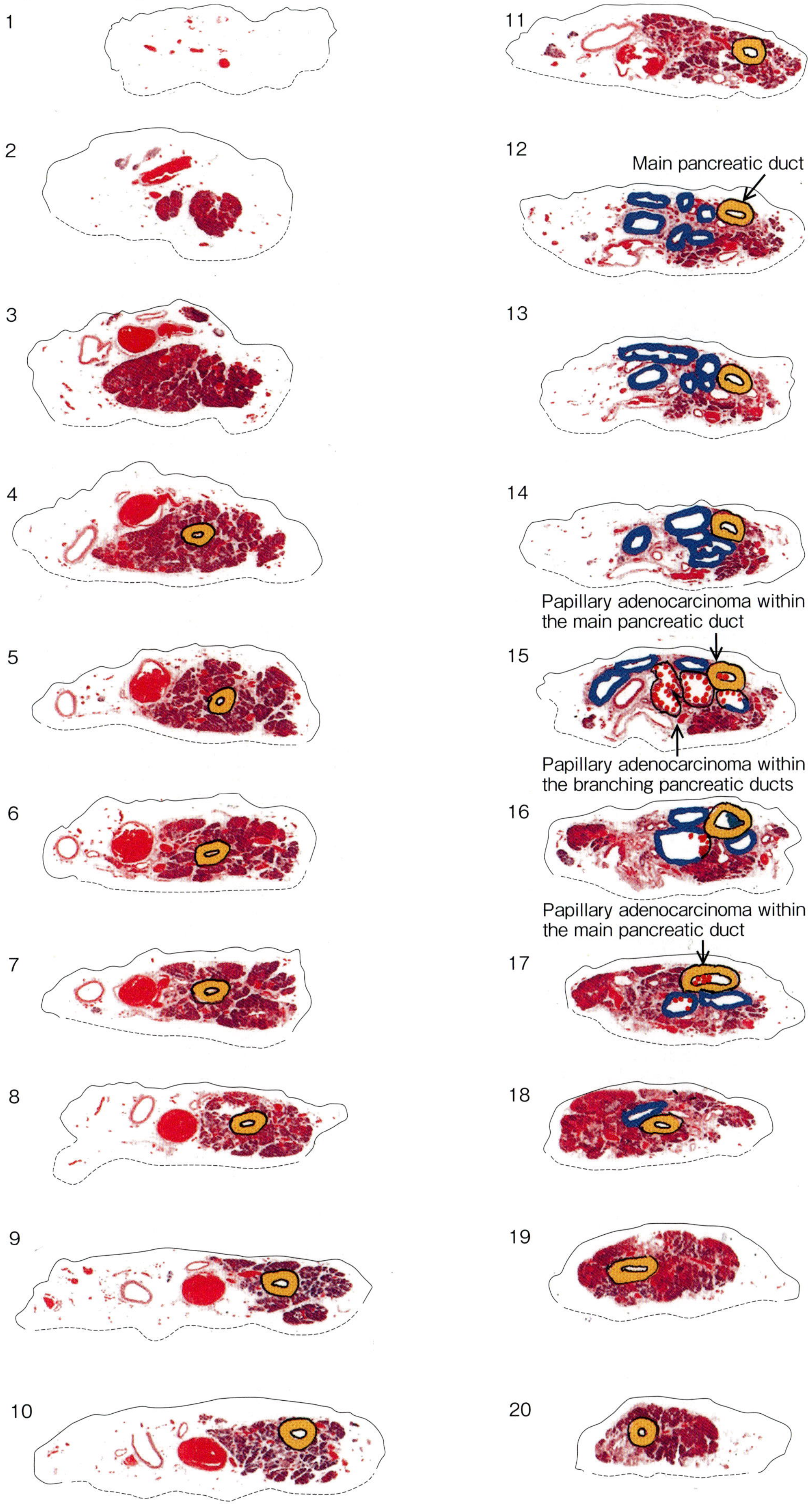

12 — Main pancreatic duct

15 — Papillary adenocarcinoma within the main pancreatic duct
Papillary adenocarcinoma within the branching pancreatic ducts

16 — Papillary adenocarcinoma within the main pancreatic duct

Red part : cancer, Blue part : adenoma

Fig. 14 Collation of the pre- and postoperative ERP images with projection views of the resected specimen

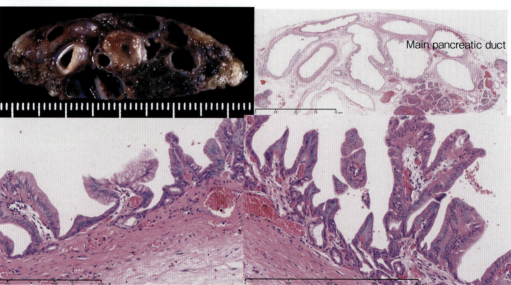

On ERP images, the primary lesion was located in Area B; the area caudad was named Area A and the area on the cranial aspect was named Area C.

Collation of the preoperative images with the histological findings

Area A : Pancreatic duct dilatation was seen, but there was no expansion of lesion. The circular region was irregular, but was histologically free of lesions.

Area B : Within the dilated main pancreatic duct and branching pancreatic ducts, there was a spread of lesions ranging from short adenomas to cancer. Identification of these papillary lesions was not possible in the images of this area.

Area C : Relatively tall papillary lesions were noted within the main pancreatic duct, and a low-density area was seen in the corresponding area of the main pancreatic duct on the ERP images.

Area B #15

a, b. A short papillary elevation was noted within the dilated main pancreatic duct and the dilated branching pancreatic ducts. c. Histological picture of the short papillary lesions seen within the branching pancreatic duct. Cellular atypia was mild, but structural atypia was marked, which led to the diagnosis of cancer. d. A short papillary lesion within the main pancreatic duct. Diagnosed as cancer because of the structural atypia.

#16

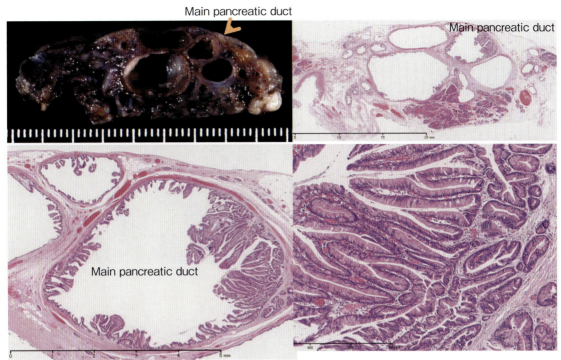

a. Photograph of the cut surface of section #16. Slightly tall papillary proliferative lesions were visible in the dilated main pancreatic duct and the dilated branching pancreatic ducts. Mucus retention was seen within the dilated pancreatic duct branches.
b, c. A macroscopically detectable papillary lesion was present in the main pancreatic duct. This site corresponded to the area denoted by the red circle on the preoperative ERP image and was visualized by preoperative radiography.
d. Magnification of the papillary lesion. On the basis of the cellular atypia and structural atypia, a diagnosis of moderately atypical adenoma was made.

Area C #17 Photograph of the cut surface

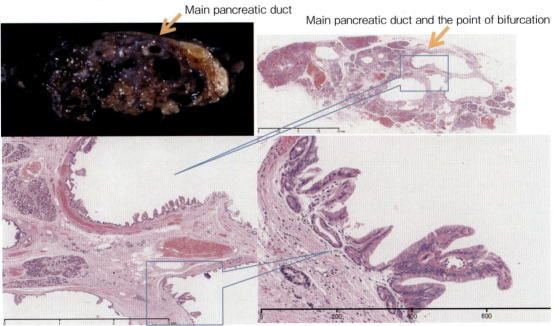

b, c. Short papillary lesions were visible within the main pancreatic duct and branching pancreatic ducts. d. Within the main pancreatic duct and the branching pancreatic ducts, lesions with mild atypia and lesions with a slightly greater degree of atypia (difficult to distinguish from cancer) had spread.

Collation of the preoperative images with the histologic features of resected specimen

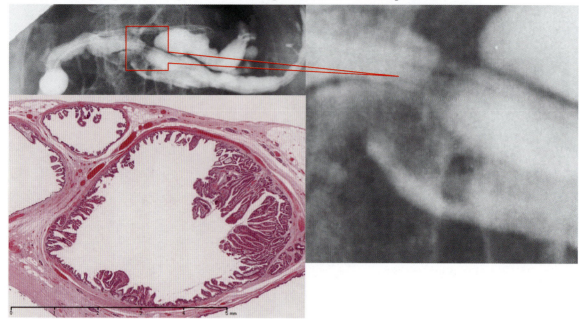

Partial stenosis seen in #16 main pancreatic duct corresponded to the slightly tall papillary proliferative lesion within the main pancreatic duct.

Histopathologic diagnosis

Intraductal papillary-mucinous neoplasm, carcinoma with adenoma, noninvasive, of the body of the pancreas
Mixed type, 50×20×7 mm, N0 (0/7)

Pathologist's comment: The papillary tumor within the wall of a dilated secondary pancreatic duct branch in the pancreatic body was a major lesion, which spread for 5 cm along the axis of the main pancreatic duct. Histologically, carcinoma in adenoma was noted in the areas showing short papillary proliferation and the areas showing flat proliferation. Because the major lesion was located in the pancreatic duct branch, we considered the macroscopic type to be "branching type", but finally decided to call it "mixed type," because a macroscopically detectable relatively large nodular lesion was also seen in the wall of the main pancreatic duct.

Clinician's comment: Clinically, judging the indication for surgery is difficult when dealing with dilated branching pancreatic ducts, as in this case. Preoperative tests in this case had revealed enlargement of the major papilla and a diameter of 9 mm of the dilated pancreatic duct branches. Endoscopic US had revealed intramural nodules, although they were short in height. We thus have an impression that in cases of non-invasive carcinoma, the mucus producing potential may be correlated with the malignancy level to some extent.

Case 4 Minimally invasive mixed-type of intraductal papillary-mucinous carcinoma (IPMC) of the pancreatic body without macroscopically detectable intramural nodule

Case: A man in his 60s
Chief complaint: Asymptomatic (lesion discovered by ultrasonography [US])
Family history: Gastric cancer in a younger sister
Past history: Tonsillectomy at age 30
Smoking and drinking history: Drinking, drank one bottle of beer/day for 45 years; smoking (−)
Present illness: In mid-January 1999, the patient underwent abdominal US as part of a health checkup at a local facility, which revealed main pancreatic duct dilatation.
He was referred to our hospital in late January 1999.
Abdominal US (Fig. 1): The main pancreatic duct was dilated extensively from the pancreatic head to the tail. There was no evident intramural nodule.
Endoscopic US (Fig. 2): Presence of an intramural nodule within the dilated main pancreatic duct in the pancreatic body region was suspected. Pancreatic duct dilatation in the pancreatic tail had extended to the branches.
Abdominal computed tomography (CT) (Fig. 3): Dilatation of the main pancreatic duct extending from the pancreatic head to the pancreatic tail, but there was no evident elevated lesion within the pancreatic duct.
Magnetic resonance cholangiopancreatography (MRCP) (Fig. 4): Dilatation of the main pancreatic duct extending from the pancreatic head to the pancreatic tail
Endoscopic findings of the duodenal papilla (Fig. 5): The opening of the major papilla was enlarged and filled with viscous mucus.
Findings on endoscopic retrograde cholangiopancreatography (ERCP) (Fig. 6): Probably because of the pooled mucus, the contrast material did not fill a part of the main pancreatic duct caudal to the pancreatic body, causing radiolucency within the pancreatic duct.
Angiography (Fig. 7): Blood vessels within the pancreas looked wavy, but there was no evident sign of encasement.
Surgical procedure (Fig. 8): In early March, caudal pancreatectomy was carried out (subtotal, operation time, 8 hours 15 minutes; blood loss, 750 g).
Macroscopic observation of the resected specimen (Fig. 9): The pancreatic body and tail were swollen, but there was no tumor exposure.
Findings on pancreatography of the resected specimen (Fig. 10): The main pancreatic duct was dilated from the pancreatic body to the tail, accompanied by cystiform dilatation of the pancreatic duct branches in the pancreatic tail region.
Findings on pancreatic duct chromoendoscopy of the resected specimen (Fig. 11): Elevated papillary lesions were noted within the main pancreatic duct, with a group of salmon roe-shaped minimal elevations seen on the surfaces of these lesions.
Postoperative course: The patient survived for 9 years after the surgery.

Blood Cell Counts	
WBC	5,000 /μL
RBC	4.18×10^6 /μL
Hb	12.8 g/dL
Ht	38.1 %
Plt	259×10^3 /μL

Tumor Markers	
CEA	1.4 ng/mL
CA19-9	34.8 U/mL
DUPAN-2	<25 U/mL
Elastase 1	270 ng/dL

Biochemistry	
TP	7.4 g/dL
T-Bil	0.56 mg/dL
γ-GTP	24 U/L
ALP	328 U/L
GOT	26 U/L
GPT	47 U/L
T-chol	216 mg/dL
Amy	53 U/L
Glu	108 mg/dL
BUN	11 mg/dL
Cre	0.56 mg/dL
Fe	83 μg/dL

I. Imaging Findings

Fig. 1 Abdominal US (transverse scanning)   **Abdominal US (pancreatic tail)**

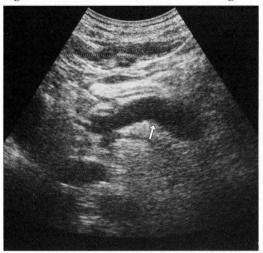 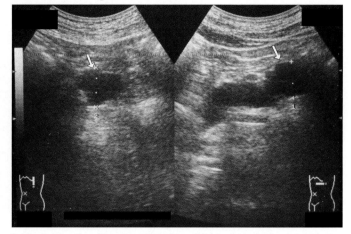

The main pancreatic duct (→) was extensively dilated from the head to the tail of the pancreas, however, there was no evident sign of an intramural nodule.

In the pancreatic tail region, dilatation of the pancreatic duct was seen to extend even into the branches (→).

Fig. 2 Endoscopic US (pancreatic body to tail)

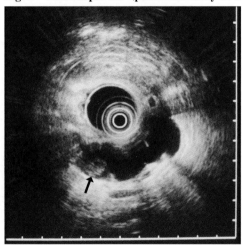 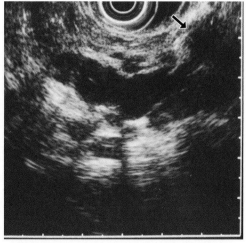

Within the dilated main pancreatic duct in the pancreatic body region, a lesion suggestive of an intramural nodule was noted (→).

In the pancreatic tail region, the dilatation of the pancreatic duct had extended even to the duct branches (→).

Fig. 3 Contrast-enhanced CT

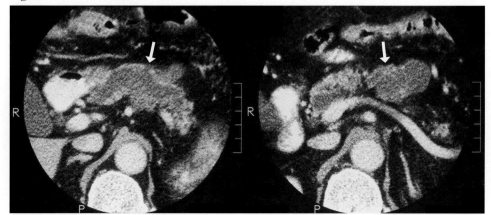

Main pancreatic duct dilatation (→) extending from the pancreatic head to the tail. There was no evident elevation within the pancreatic duct.

Fig. 4 MRCP

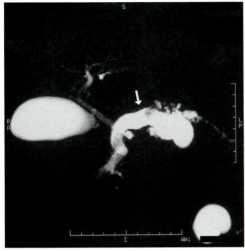

Main pancreatic duct dilatation (→) extending from the head to the tail

Fig. 5 Endoscopic findings of the duodenal papilla

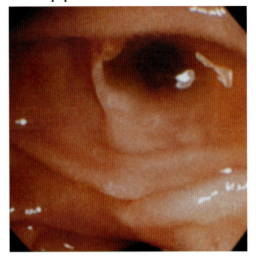

The opening of the major papilla was enlarged and filled with viscous mucus.

Fig. 6 Endoscopic retrograde pancreatography (ERP)

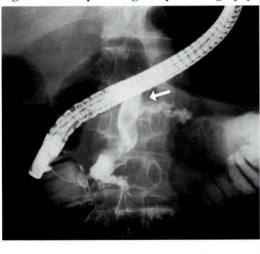 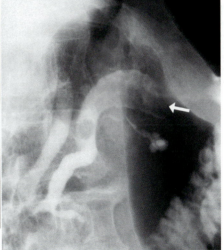

Probably because of the pooled mucus, the contrast material did not fill a part of the main pancreatic duct caudal to the pancreatic body (→), causing a radiolucency within the pancreatic duct.

Fig. 7 Angiography

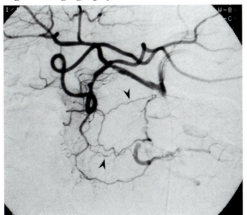

Blood vessels within the pancreas looked wavy (▶), but there was no evident sign of encasement.

II. Surgical Findings

Fig. 8 Surgical findings

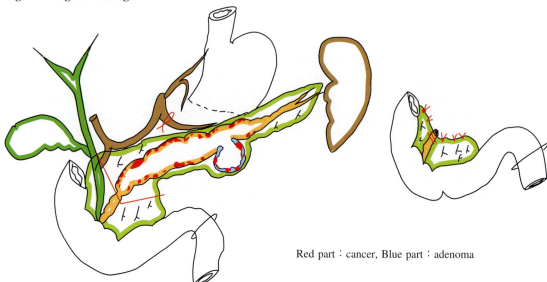

Red part : cancer, Blue part : adenoma

Fig. 9 Close observation of the anterior plane of the resected specimen

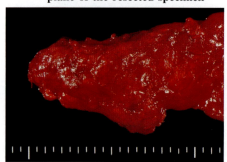

The pancreatic body and tail were swollen, but there was no exposed tumor.

Fig. 10 Pancreatography of the resected specimen

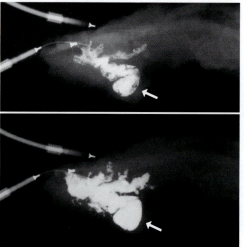

The main pancreatic duct was dilated in the pancreatic body and tail regions, accompanied by cystic dilatation of the pancreatic duct branches in the tail region (→).

Fig. 11 Pancreatic duct chromoendoscopy of the resected specimen

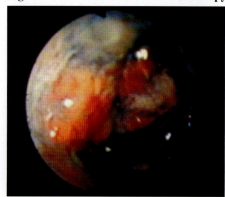

There were elevated papillary lesions within the main pancreatic duct.

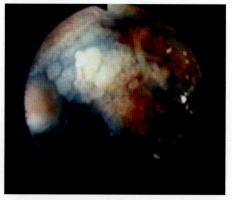

A group of small salmon roe-shaped elevations were visible on the surfaces of the elevated lesions.

III. Pathological Findings

Fig. 12 Tissue architecture of the resected specimen

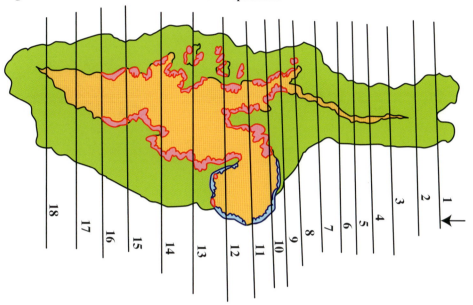

Red part : cancer, Blue part : adenoma

Fig. 13 Findings of the cut surfaces of the resected specimen

1. Findings of the cut surfaces of all the sections of the resected specimen

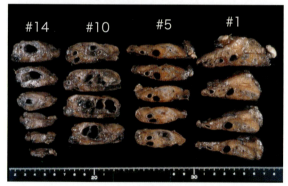

2. Findings of the cut surfaces of sections #10 to 14

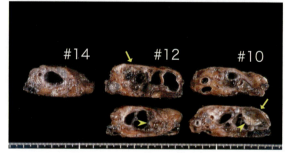

Within the dilated main pancreatic duct and pancreatic duct branches, mucus-filled areas (→) and a nodular elevations (➤) were seen sporadically.

3. Findings of the cut surface of section #11

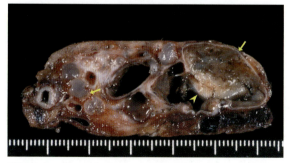

Within the dilated main pancreatic duct and pancreatic duct branches, mucus-filled areas (→) and a nodular elevation (➤) were seen sporadically.

4. Findings of the cut surface of section #12

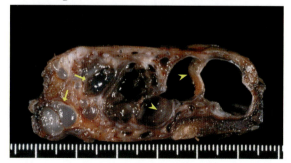

Within the dilated main pancreatic duct and pancreatic duct branches, mucus-filled areas (→) and nodular elevations (➤) were seen sporadically.

48

Fig. 14 Findings of the cut surfaces of all the sections of the resected specimen

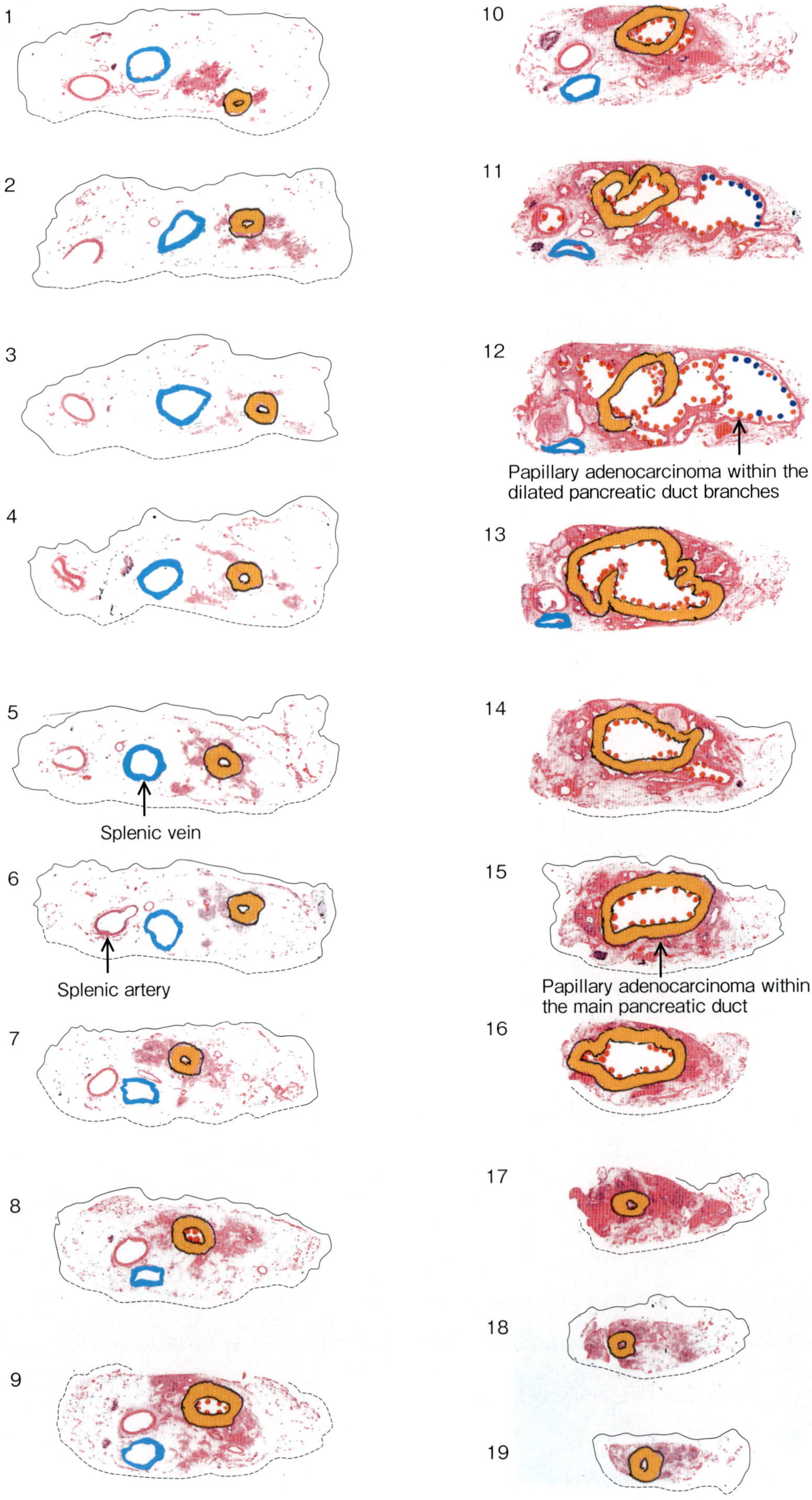

1
2
3
4
5 Splenic vein
6 Splenic artery
7
8
9
10
11
12 Papillary adenocarcinoma within the dilated pancreatic duct branches
13
14
15 Papillary adenocarcinoma within the main pancreatic duct
16
17
18
19

Red part : cancer, Blue part : adenoma

Fig. 15 Collation of the preoperative ERCP/magnetic resonance imaging (MRI) images and postoperative ERP images with projection views of the resected specimen

Preoperative ERCP

Preoperative magnetic resonance perfusion (MRP) images

Postoperative ERP images

Comparison with the projection view

It was difficult to determine the location of the cystic dilatation (in the main pancreatic duct or in the pancreatic duct branches), however, the postoperative image projections showed that the dilatation was centered in the pancreatic duct branches. Among the preoperative images, MRP images allowed it to be judged that the dilatation had begun in the pancreatic duct branches.

Histological features of the lesions are shown for Area A (free of dilatation of the main pancreatic duct in the pancreatic tail region), Area B (with dilatation of the duct), Area C (with dilatation of the main pancreatic duct and pancreatic duct branches) and Area D (with dilatation of the main pancreatic duct in the pancreatic head).

Area A : Histological features
#5 Loupe image (atrophy of the pancreatic parenchyma)

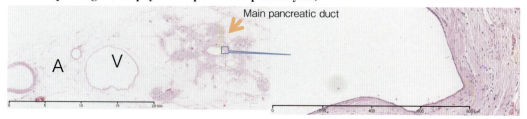

Marked atrophy of the pancreatic parenchyma and slight dilatation of the main pancreatic duct were visible, but the epithelium consisted of a layer of atypia-free flat epithelial cells.

Area B #9

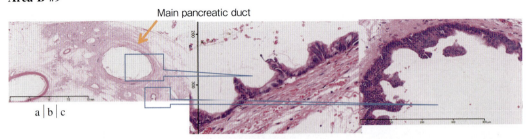

a. Loupe image of the dilated part of the main pancreatic duct. b. A short papillary lesion that was not visible macroscopically as a papillary lesion. Cancer with strong cellular atypia had spread along the full circumference of the main pancreatic duct lumen. c. Spread of cancer with similar histological features was also seen within the pancreatic duct branches.

Area C

#11

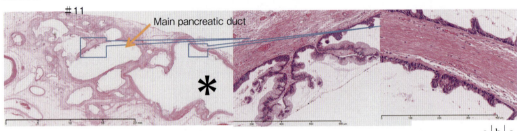

a. Numerous dilated pancreatic ducts were visible. There was no macroscopically visible nodular elevated lesion on the pancreatic duct wall. b, c. Histologically, cancer showing short papillary proliferation had spread in the main pancreatic duct and pancreatic duct branches. The relatively tall papillary proliferative lesion was diagnosed as an adenoma.

＊Corresponding to the pancreatic duct branches showing cystic dilatation on the ERP/MRP images (Fig. 15)

#12

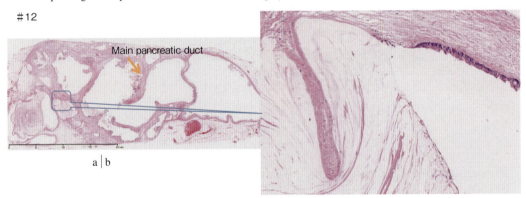

a. The wall of the dilated pancreatic duct was mostly flat when viewed macroscopically. Histologically, the wall epithelium was composed of flat or short papillary lesions, including cancer and adenoma lesions. b. The wall of the pancreatic duct branch was partially destroyed, resulting in outflow of mucus into the stroma. Because the mucus did not contain cancer cells, it was doubtful if invasion had occurred. However, because the mucus was produced by the cancer, a judgment of invasion was made. The extent of invasion was regarded as minimal, because only mucinous nodules were found.

Area D

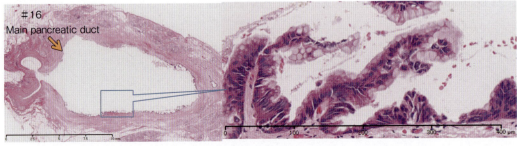

Spread of cancer was also seen to the cranial segment of the dilated main pancreatic duct. Cancer spread was seen in specimens up to #16. The pancreatic duct cranial to this point was, however, cancer-free.

Collation of the preoperative images with projection views of the resected specimen

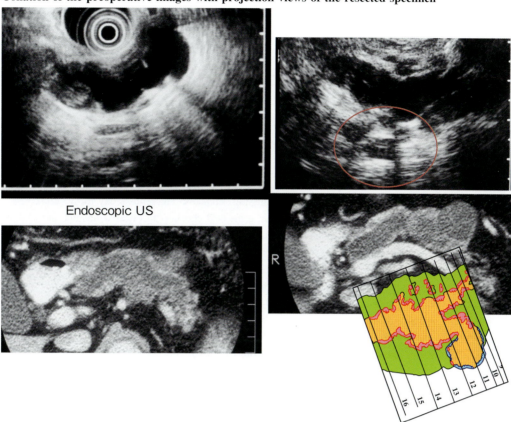

In the wall of the dilated pancreatic duct seen on the diagnostic images, cancer spread was confirmed histologically, even though the diagnosis of cancer spread was difficult on the basis of diagnostic imaging alone. The endoscopic ultrasound image suggesting the presence of an intramural nodule was likely to reflect a mucinous nodule, because histological examination revealed no tall papillary proliferative lesion.

Histopathologic diagnosis

Intraductal papillary-mucinous neoplasm (IPMN), carcinoma with adenoma, minimally invasive, of the body and tail of the pancreas
Mixed type, 60×40×20 mm, N0 (0/7)

Pathologist's comment: This is a case of a pancreatic body IPMN, almost free of nodular lesions. The tumor had spread extensively on the wall of the dilated main pancreatic duct and pancreatic duct branches. Within the wall, there was no macroscopically visible tall nodular lesion. The epithelium which had grown within the wall contained diverse lesions, ranging from strongly atypical cancer to adenoma. The pancreatic duct wall was partially destroyed, apparently as a result of 'falling off' of the mucinous nodules. Thus, a diagnosis of minimally invasive cancer was made.

Clinician's comment: Extensive dilatation of the main pancreatic duct and pancreatic duct branches was seen, primarily in the pancreatic body region, however, diagnostic imaging did not reveal the presence of any significant elevated lesion within the pancreatic duct. The tumor was clinically rated as having a high mucus-producing potential, however, the tumor within the pancreatic duct was histopathologically confirmed to show short papillary proliferation to flat proliferation. Nine years have passed after subtotal caudal pancreatectomy in this case. At present, diagnostic imaging shows no abnormalities in the residual pancreas.

Case 5 Branch duct-type non-invasive intraductal papillary-mucinous carcinoma (IPMC) with concurrent carcinoma in situ (CIS) at three sites

Case: A woman in her 60s
Chief complaint: Asymptomatic (lesion discovered by ultrasonography [US])
Family history: No history of cancer
Past history: A cesarean section at age 26 and an operation for myoma uteri at age 45
Smoking and drinking history: Drinking (−); smoking, smoked 5 cigarettes a day for 30 years
Present illness: In late February 1998, she underwent a medical checkup at a nearby hospital and abdominal US revealed dilatation of the main pancreatic duct.
On the same day, she was admitted to another hospital for further evaluation, and an intraductal tumor of the main pancreatic duct in the head of the pancreas was diagnosed.
The patient was first seen at our hospital in mid-March.
Abdominal US (Fig. 1): Dilatation of the main pancreatic duct in the head of the pancreas (closer to the body of the pancreas) and also of the adjacent pancreatic duct branches
Endosonographic examination (Fig. 2): Small agminate cysts were seen in the head of the pancreas.
Contrast-enhanced computed tomography (CT) of the abdomen (Fig. 3): Small agminate cysts and dilatation of the main pancreatic duct were noted in the head of the pancreas.
Endoscopic findings of the duodenal papilla (Fig. 4): There was no widening of the orifice of the papilla of Vater.
Findings of endoscopic retrograde cholangiopancreatography (ERCP) (Fig. 5): The main pancreatic duct was dilated, mainly at the pancreatic head-body junction, with some dilation, irregular lumina and radiolucencies of adjacent branches of the pancreatic duct.
Surgical procedure (Fig. 6): In mid-April, a pylorus-preserving pancreaticoduodenectomy was performed (operation time, 12 hours 40 minutes; blood loss, 720 g).
Intraoperative pancreatoscopic findings (Fig. 7): The main pancreatic duct epithelium was coarse, with red plaques and dilation of the blood vessels seen within the duct. A small nodular elevation was also observed within the duct.
Findings on the anterior aspect of the resected specimen (Fig. 8): There was no tumor exposure on the anterior aspect of the head of the pancreas.
Pancreatographic findings of the resected specimen (Fig. 9): The main pancreatic duct in the head of the pancreas was dilated and dilatation and radiolucency of the duct branch were also seen at the pancreatic head-body junction.
Postoperative course: The patient survived for 5 years after the surgery.

Blood Cell Counts	
WBC	6,600 /μL
RBC	3.90×10^6 /μL
Hb	12.9 g/dL
Ht	37.3 %
Plt	195×10^3 /μL

Tumor Markers	
CEA	2.0 ng/mL
CA19-9	0.6 U/mL
DUPAN-2	<25 U/mL
Elastase 1	140 ng/dL

Biochemistry	
TP	7.3 g/dL
Alb	4.7 g/dL
T-Bil	0.7 mg/dL
γ-GTP	36 U/L
ALP	199 U/L
GOT	21 U/L
GPT	26 U/L
Amy	146 U/L
P-Amy	88 U/L
Glu	105 mg/dL
BUN	9 mg/dL
Crea	0.70 mg/dL

I. Imaging Findings

Fig. 1 Abdominal US

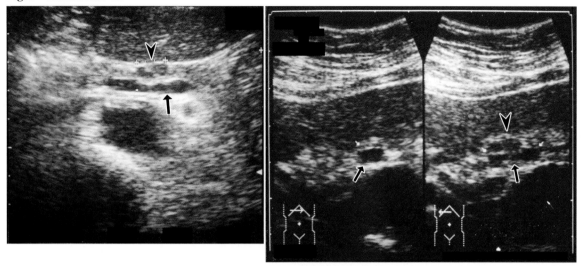

Dilatation of the main pancreatic duct was observed in the head of the pancreas (closer to the body of the pancreas) (→) and dilatation of the adjacent pancreatic duct branches was also observed (➤).

Fig. 2 Endosonographic examination

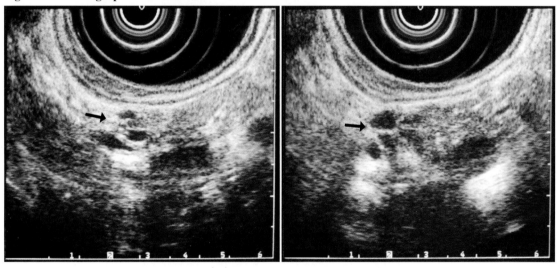

Small cysts (→) were seen in the head of the pancreas.

Fig. 3 Contrast-enhanced CT

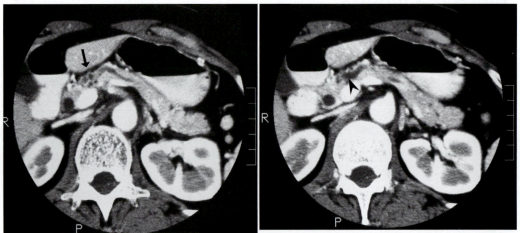

Small cysts (→) and dilatation of the main pancreatic duct (➤) were noted in the head of the pancreas.

Fig. 4 Endoscopy of the duodenal papilla

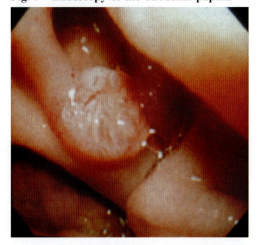

There was no widening of the orifice of the papilla of Vater.

Fig. 5 ERCP

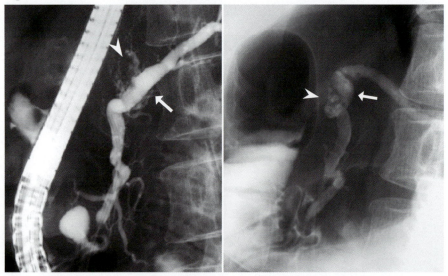

The main pancreatic duct was dilated, mainly at the pancreatic head-body junction (→), with some dilation, irregular lumina and radiolucencies (➤) of the adjacent pancreatic duct branches.

II. Surgical Findings

Fig. 6 Surgical findings

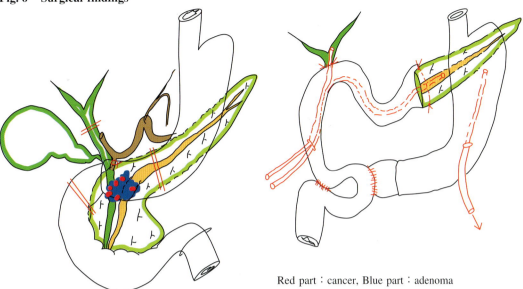

Red part : cancer, Blue part : adenoma

Fig. 7 Intraoperative pancreatoscopy

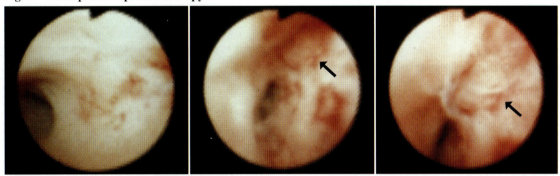

Endoscopic examination of the main pancreatic duct from the stump revealed a coarse epithelium, red plaques and dilated blood vessels along with a small nodular elevation (→).

Fig. 8 Resected specimen (anterior view)

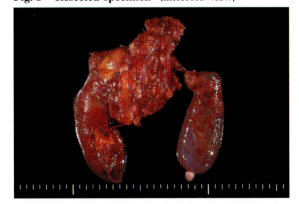

There was no tumor exposure on the anterior aspect of the head of the pancreas.

Fig. 9 Pancreatogram of the resected specimen

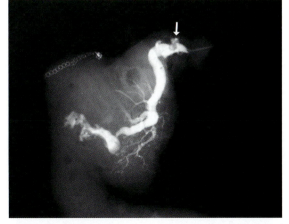

Examination of the main pancreatic duct after injection of contrast into the stump of the pancreas revealed dilatation of the main pancreatic duct in the head of the pancreas, with dilatation and radiolucency (→) of the pancreatic duct branches at the pancreatic head-body junction.

III. Pathological Findings

Fig. 10 Tissue architecture of the resected specimen

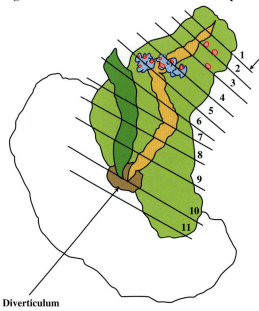

Red part：cancer
Blue part：adenoma

Diverticulum

Fig. 11 Findings of the cut surfaces of the resected specimen

1. Findings of the cut surfaces of all sections of the resected specimen

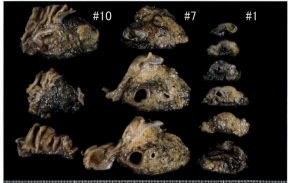

2. Findings of cut surfaces of sections #3 to 5

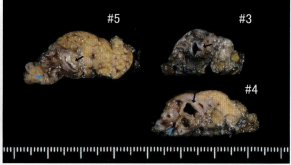

The main pancreatic duct was dilated (→), surrounded by dilated agminate pancreatic duct branches (►).

3. Findings of the cut surface of section #4

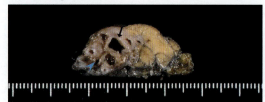

The main pancreatic duct was dilated (→), surrounded by dilated agminate pancreatic duct branches (►).

4. Findings of the front cut surface of section #5

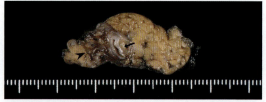

The main pancreatic duct was dilated (→), surrounded by dilated agminate pancreatic duct branches (►).

5. Findings on the rear cut surface of section #5

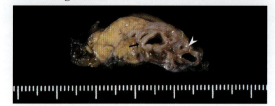

The main pancreatic duct was dilated (→), surrounded by dilated agminate pancreatic duct branches (►).

Case 5 Branch duct-type non-invasive intraductal papillary-mucinous carcinoma (IPMC) with concurrent carcinoma in situ (CIS) at three sites

Fig. 12 Findings of the cut surfaces of all sections of the resected specimen

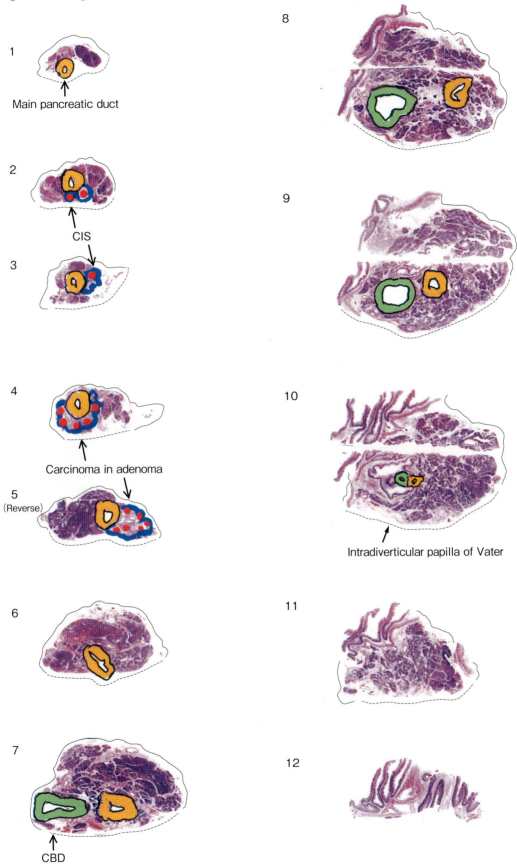

Red part: cancer, Blue part: adenoma

Fig. 13 Collation of the pre- and postoperative endoscopic retrograde pancreatography (ERP) images with projection views of the postoperative specimen

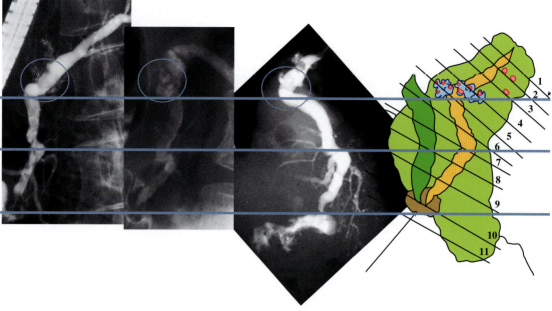

Red part : cancer, Blue part : adenoma
Correlated by matching the orifice of the papilla and the convoluted main pancreatic duct
Pre- and postoperative ERP images : The main pancreatic duct was dilated, along with dilatation and radiolucency (blue circle) also of a pancreatic duct branch at the head-body junction.

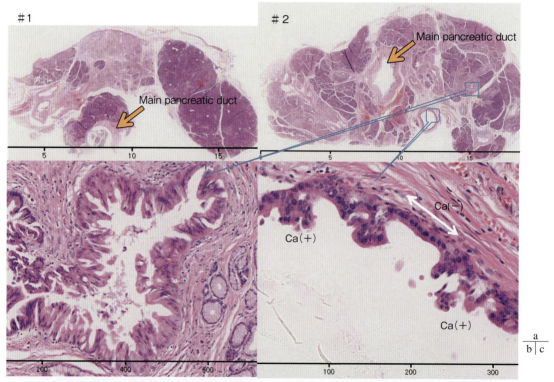

#1 The main pancreatic duct was noted. There was no tumorous lesion in the pancreatic duct wall.
#2 Dilatation of the main pancreatic duct and also of an adjacent pancreatic duct branch was seen. There was no tumorous lesion in the main pancreatic duct, however, discontinuous short papillary lesions were noted at two sites of the pancreatic duct branch wall epithelium. b, c. A diagnosis of cellular-atypical, structural atypia-like carcinoma was made, although differentiation between carcinoma and strongly atypical adenoma was needed. A diagnosis of carcinoma was made in this case, since stump recurrence was very likely to occur if such a lesion was evident at the stump and since continuity with a site of invasion was often seen. c. Showing the border between the noncancerous region and the cancer

#3

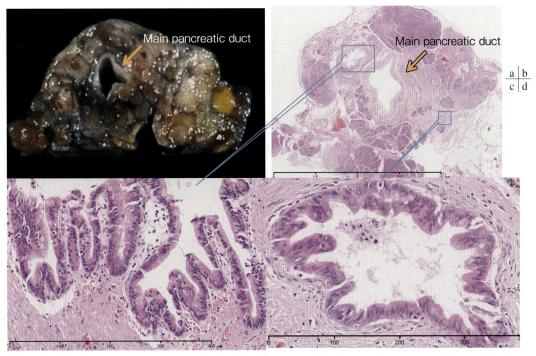

a, b. A dilated main pancreatic duct surrounded by dilated branches of the duct. c. There was a papillary proliferative lesion in the wall of a duct branch. Moderate cellular and structural atypia was seen, and a diagnosis of moderately atypical adenoma was made. No atypical lesion was noted in the main pancreatic duct. d. A peripheral pancreatic duct branch had atypical epithelium with severe cellular/structural atypia. This atypical epithelium was not continuous with the atypical epithelium seen in section #2; therefore, multiple atypical epithelium was diagnosed.

#4

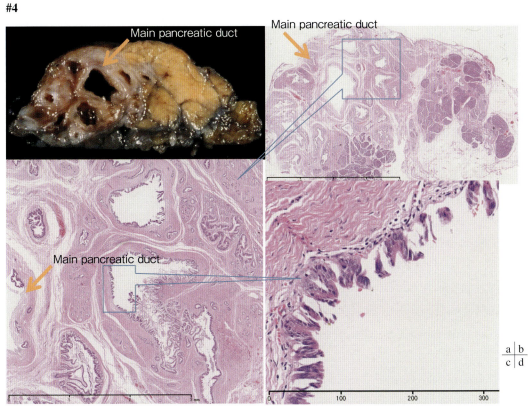

a, b. The main pancreatic duct and a duct branch were dilated. b, c. Papillary proliferative lesions were seen in the duct branch. d. A diagnosis of carcinoma was made on account of the severe cellular/structural atypia of the epithelium of the duct branch.

Collation of the pre- and postoperative images of essentially the same sites with those on the postoperative resected specimen

Contrast-enhanced CT findings   Endosonographic findings

As there was a progressive carcinoma with short papillary proliferative lesions was seen in the pancreatic duct branch, intraductal carcinoma of a duct branch should be carefully diagnosed on ERP.

Histopathologic diagnosis

Carcinoma in situ (3 sites) and intraductal papillary-mucinous neoplasm, carcinoma in adenoma (triple CISs and IPMC)

1. Intraductal papillary-mucinous neoplasm, carcinoma in adenoma, non-invasive
   Branch type, 20×10×10 mm, N0 (0/18)
2. Triple CISs in the head of the pancreas

Pathologist's comment : Lesions were noted primarily in the wall of the dilated pancreatic duct branches. For the most part, the lesions were diagnosed as adenoma with modest atypia, and there were non-invasive carcinoma components sporadically within the adenoma. In addition, carcinoma in situ entirely non-continuous with the major lesion was noted at 3 sites.

Clinician's comment : Preoperative diagnostic imaging examinations revealed circumscribed dilatation of the main pancreatic duct in the head of the pancreas, with adjacent multilocular cysts. The cytology grade of the pancreatic juice collected intraoperatively from the main pancreatic duct was Class V.

Case 6 Invasive carcinoma derived from branch-duct type intraductal papillary-mucinous neoplasm (IPMN): A case with inferred transition to invasive carcinoma during a 5-year follow-up course

Case: A woman in her 70s

Chief complaint: Asymptomatic (lesion discovered by computed tomography [CT]. Patient followed up for 5 years and 6 months)

Family history: No family history of cancer

Past history: Cholecystectomy for a gallbladder polyp (hyperplasia) at our hospital at age 63

Smoking and drinking history: Drinking (−); smoking (−)

Present illness: In April 1999, a CT performed as part of a follow-up post-cholecystecomy revealed an 8-mm cystic lesion at the border between the head and body of the pancreas. She continued to be kept under observation by periodic checkups thereafter. Her serum CA19-9 level was 27.4 U/mL at that time. At subsequent once-yearly checkups, the cystic lesion remained unchanged on the CT images, and there was no noticeable change of the serum CA19-9 values (U/mL), i.e., 32.2 (2000)→32.7 (2001)→24.4 (2002). In March 2004, however, the diameter of the lesion in the head of the pancreas had increased to 10 mm and the shape of the lesion had changed on imaging. As there was also an increase of the serum CA19-9 level to 94.0 U/mL, the patient was advised surgery, but refused.

In October 2004, the lesion diameter had increased to 15 mm in the major axis and changed further in shape. The serum CA19-9 value had increased to 160.1 U/mL.

Abdominal Ultrasonography over time (Fig. 1): The cystic lesion in the head of the pancreas (close to the pancreatic body), which was 8 mm in diameter at the checkup conducted in March 2001, had become a large mass measuring 23 mm in diameter with internal homogeneous echoes in October 2004.

Endosonographic examination (Fig. 2): A hypoechoic mass, 20 mm in its major axis, was detected in the head of the pancreas (close to the pancreatic body).

Contrast-enhanced CT of the abdomen over time (Fig. 3): The cystic lesion in the head of the pancreas (close to the pancreatic body) that was 8 mm in diameter at the checkup conducted in April 2001 began to show contraction in size with expansion of a pericystic low-intensity area from 2003. In October 2004, the lesion increased to 20 mm in its major axis, with the cyst contracted and filled with a low-intensity solid pattern.

Endoscopic retrograde cholangiopancreatography (ERCP) images and endoscopic findings of the duodenal papilla over time (Fig. 4): The orifice of the papilla of Vater was slightly open, but no marked changes were observed from March to October 2004.

ERCP findings (Fig. 4): In March 2004, extramural compression stenosis of the main pancreatic duct was noted in the head of the pancreas (close to the pancreatic body). By October 2004, the stenosis had progressed, along with conspicuous distension of the main pancreatic duct in the tail region of the pancreas.

Findings on endoscopic retrograde pancreatography (ERP)-CT (by maximum intensity projection [MIP]) (Fig. 4): The cystic region around the stenosed segment of the main pancreatic duct contracted in size over the 7-month period from March to October 2004.

Surgical procedure (Fig. 5): In mid-December 2004, subtotal stomach-preserving pancreaticoduodenectomy was performed (operation time, 8 hours 7 minutes; blood loss, 180 g).

Findings at the anterior aspect of resected specimen (Fig. 6): There was no tumor exposure on the anterior aspect of the head-to-body of the pancreas.

Pancreatographic findings of the resected specimen (Fig. 7): The main pancreatic duct in the head of the pancreas (close to the pancreatic body) showed a stenosed segment about 15 mm in length, with dilatation of the duct in the caudal aspect.

Postoperative course: The patient survived for 7 years 8 months after the surgery.

Blood Cell Counts		Biochemistry	
WBC	4,900 /μL	TP	7.1 g/dL
RBC	3.80×10⁶ /μL	T-Bil	0.7 mg/dL
Hb	11.6 g/dL	γ-GTP	24 U/L
Ht	35.1 %	ALP	189 U/L
Plt	206×10³ /mL	GOT	24 U/L
		GPT	17 U/L
Tumor Markers		T-chol	219 mg/dL
CEA	2.0 ng/mL	Amy	123 U/L
CA19-9	160.1 U/mL	Glu	106 mg/dL
DUPAN-2	<25 U/mL	BUN	14 mg/dL
Elastase 1	290 ng/dL	Crea	0.60 mg/dL
		Fe	95 mg/dL

I. Imaging Findings

Fig. 1 Abdominal ultrasonography

1. March 2001

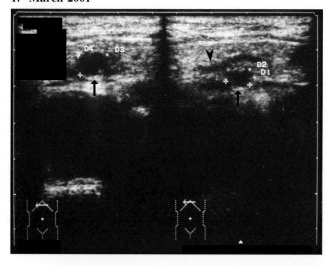

Two cystic lesions (→) measuring 8 mm in their major axes were seen in the head of the pancreas (close to the pancreatic body) adjacent to each other in the vicinity of the main pancreatic duct (►).

2. October 2004

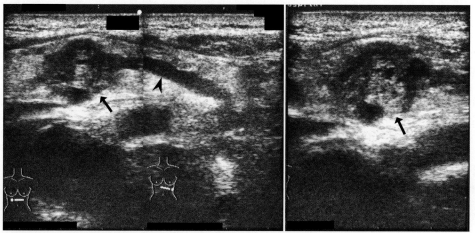

There was a round hypoechoic mass measuring 23 mm in its major axis (→) in the head of the pancreas (close to the pancreatic body), with an internal nonhomogeneous echo pattern. The main pancreatic duct (►) caudad to this lesion was dilated.

Fig. 2 Endosonography (October 2004)

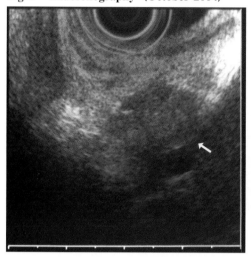

A hypoechoic mass measuring 20 mm in its major axis (→) was seen in the head of the pancreas (close to the pancreatic body).

Fig. 3 Findings on contrast-enhanced CT over time

1. April 2001
2. March 2002
3. March 2003
4. March 2004

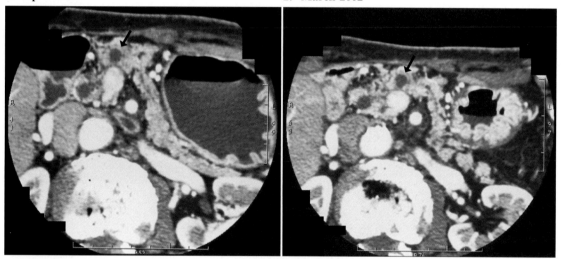

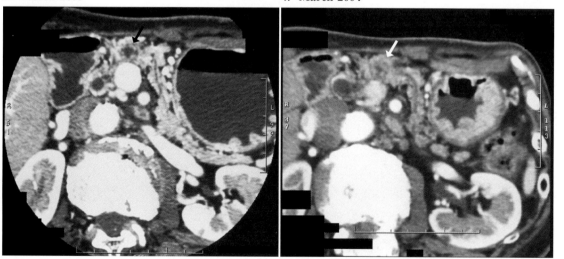

The cyst component of the cystic lesion (→) in the head of the pancreas had contracted progressively from 2003 with an expanding pericystic low-density area.

5. October 2004

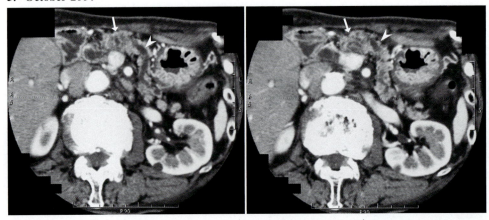

The cystic lesion (→) in the head of the pancreas (close to the pancreatic body) had increased in size to 2 cm in its major axis, with contraction of the cyst filled with a low-density solid pattern. The main pancreatic duct caudad to the mass was dilated (▶).

Fig. 4 1. ERCP (March 2004)

ERP   Endoscopic findings of the papilla of Vater   ERP-CT (by MIP)

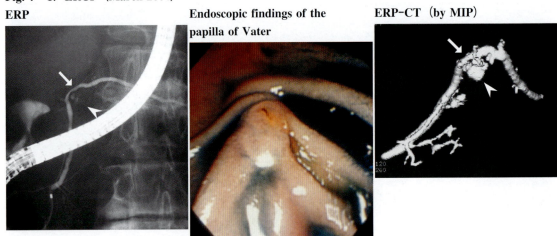

The orifice of the major duodenal papilla was slightly open. Compression stenosis of the main pancreatic duct (→) was noted in the head of the pancreas (close to the pancreatic body), along with accumulation of contrast medium (▶) in its vicinity.

2. ERP (October 2004)

ERP   Endoscopic findings of the papilla of Vater   ERP-CT (by MIP)

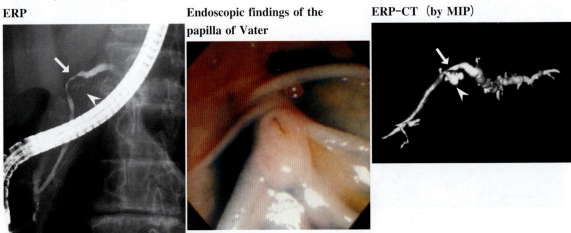

There was no remarkable change in the orifice of the papilla of Vater. The main pancreatic duct stenosis (→) had progressed further in 7 months and the distension of the main pancreatic duct caudad to stenotic segment was conspicuous. The decrease in contrast medium accumulation (▶) in the vicinity was considered to reflect the contraction of the cyst.

II. Surgical Findings

Fig. 5 Surgical findings

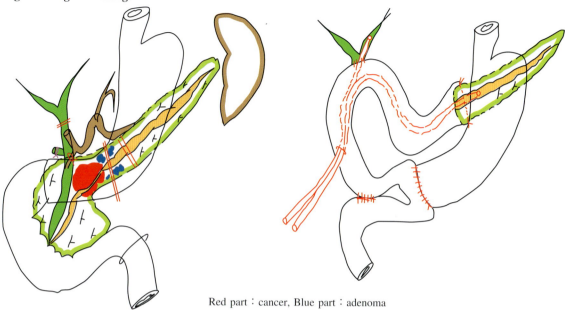

Red part : cancer, Blue part : adenoma

Fig. 6 Resected specimen (anterior aspect)

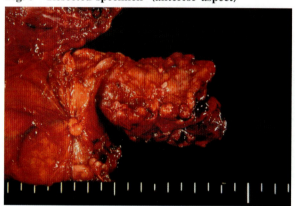

There was no tumor exposure on the anterior aspect of the pancreas, anywhere from the head to the body.

Fig. 7 Findings on pancreatocholangiography of the resected specimen

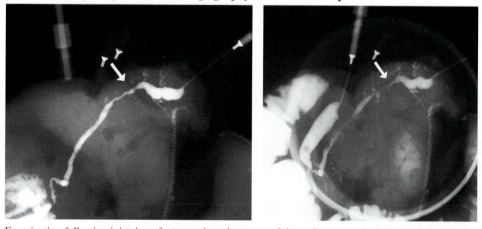

Examination following injection of contrast into the stump of the main pancreatic duct revealed a stenotic segment of the main pancreatic duct in the head of the pancreas (close to the pancreatic body) (→) measuring about 1.5 cm in length, with dilatation of the duct caudad to this segment. The contrast medium retention in the vicinity of the stenosed segment, which was noted on the ERP, was no longer existent.

III. Pathological Findings

Fig. 8　Tissue architecture of the resected specimen

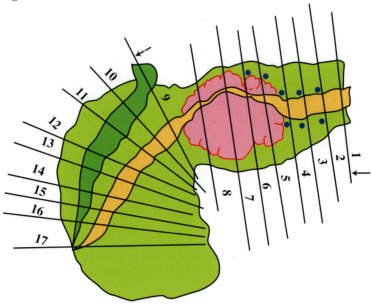

Red part : cancer, Blue part : adenoma

Fig. 9　Findings of the cut surfaces of the resected specimen

1. Photograph of the cut surfaces of all sections of the resected specimen

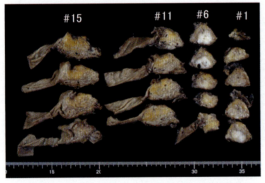

2. Photograph of the cut surfaces of sections #5 and 6

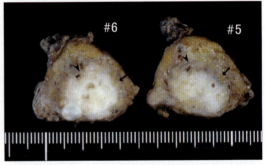

A grayish-white nodular mass measuring 28 mm in its major axis (→) was noted dorsal to the main pancreatic duct (▶) in the head of the pancreas (close to the pancreatic body), and microcysts were seen in the mass.

3. Photograph of the cut surfaces of sections #7 and 8

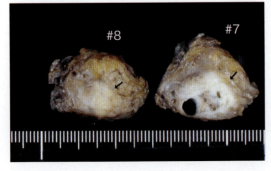

There was a grayish-white nodular mass (→) situated dorsally in the head of the pancreas (close to the pancreatic body) with microcysts in the mass.

Fig. 10 Findings of the cut surfaces of all sections of the resected specimen

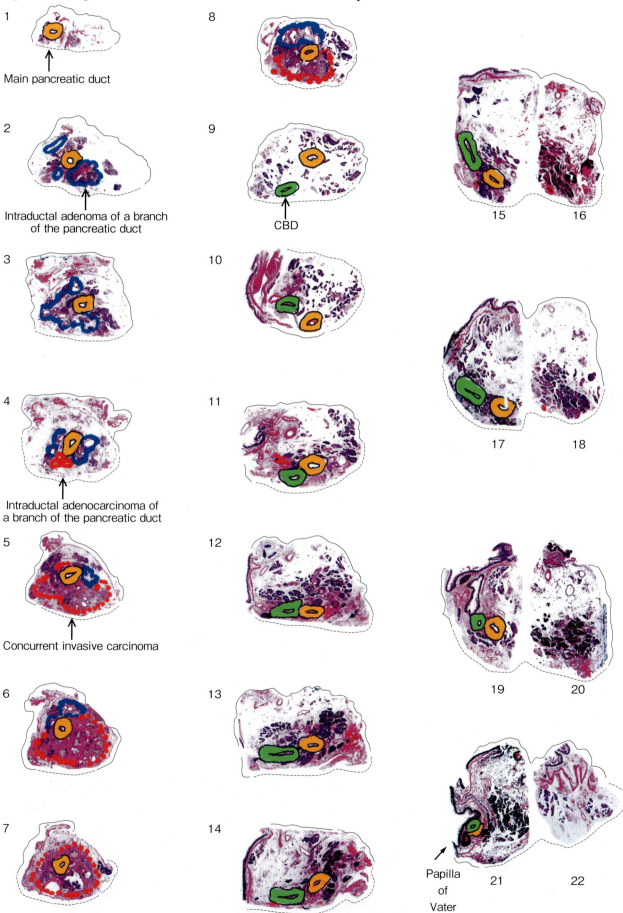

Fig. 11 Collation of the pre- and postoperative ERP and ERP-CT (by MIP) images with projection views of the resected specimen

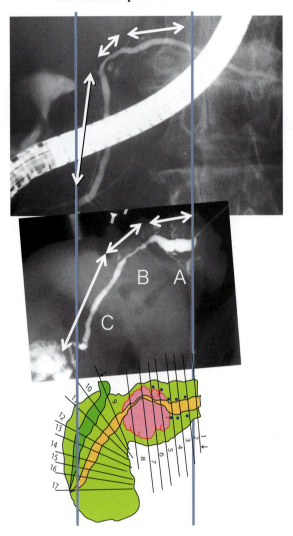
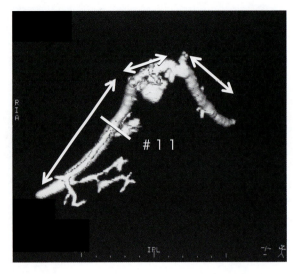

The correlation of the pre- and postoperative images with the projection views was carried out with respect to the main part of the lesion and the B region.
Correlated by matching the orifice of the papilla of Vater and stump of the resection

B region #4

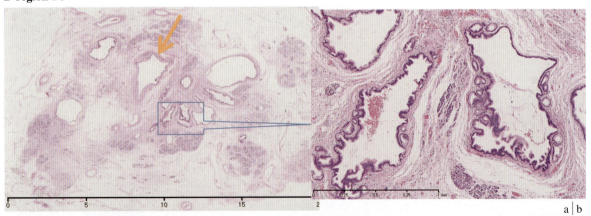

a. A slightly dilated main pancreatic duct (arrow) and many dilated pancreatic duct branches were seen. b. There were low papillary proliferative lesions in the epithelium of the pancreatic duct branches. The lesion was diagnosed as an adenoma on account of the modest atypia of the component cells and mild structural atypia. There was no progression of the lesion in the main pancreatic duct.

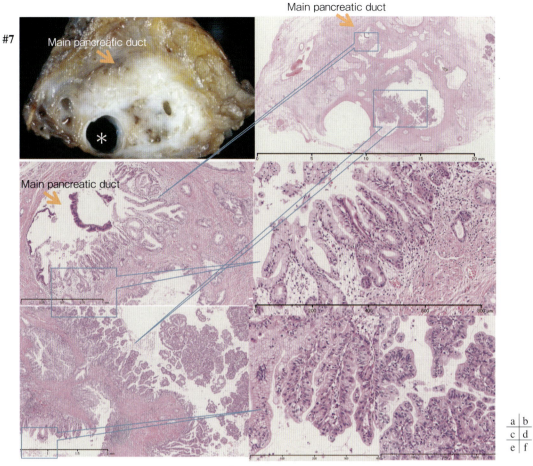

a, b, c. Section showing the main pancreatic duct (arrow) and bifurcation of a pancreatic duct branch. It was noted that the progressing carcinoma in the dilated branch was continuous with the carcinoma in the main pancreatic duct, as evident even on this section alone. c, d. These photomicrographs showed progression of the carcinoma represented by the low papillary proliferation in the wall of the main pancreatic duct. Invasive carcinoma was noted in the perimural region, where there was no continuity between the intramural carcinoma and the invasive carcinoma. d, e, f. These photomicrographs showed progression of the carcinoma represented by papillary proliferation in the wall of the dilated branch of the pancreatic duct. The carcinoma was composed of cells with mucus-rich cytoplasm and cells with relatively mucus-poor cytoplasm, and continuity was observed between the two.
＊The dilated cyst was a retention cyst.

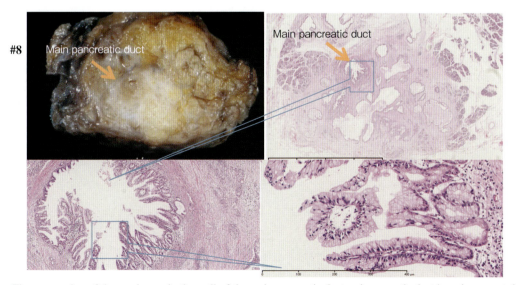

The progression of the carcinoma in the wall of the main pancreatic duct and pancreatic duct branch was noted.

Collation between the pre- and postoperative pancreatograms and projection views of the resected specimen

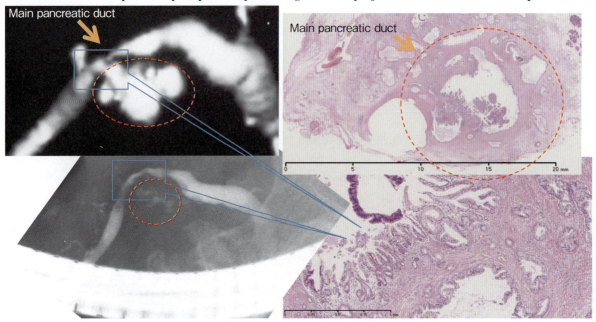

Collation between the photomicrographs and pancreatographic images of the regions corresponding to the main pancreatic duct and bifurcation of a pancreatic duct branch. Progressing infiltrative carcinoma in the walls of the main pancreatic duct and branch of the pancreatic duct was encompassed in part by a red dotted circle.

There was progression of cancer in the epithelium of the stenosed segment of the main pancreatic duct in the ERP image, where the irregularity of the wall of the main pancreatic duct was suggestive of malignancy.

April 2001   **March 2004**

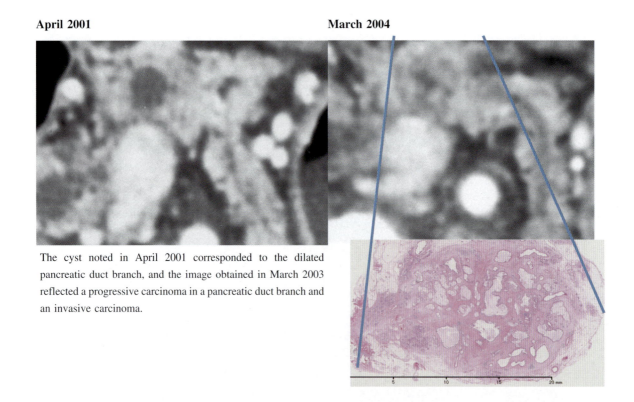

The cyst noted in April 2001 corresponded to the dilated pancreatic duct branch, and the image obtained in March 2003 reflected a progressive carcinoma in a pancreatic duct branch and an invasive carcinoma.

Histopathologic diagnosis

Intraductal papillary-mucinous neoplasm, carcinoma with adenoma, invasive, of the head of the pancreas
Branch type, 25×20×14 mm, INFb, ly0, v0, ne1, pw (−), ew (−), N0 (0/6)

Pathologist's comment: Changes were noted primarily in the lumen and wall of the dilated pancreatic duct branches, with slight involvement of the wall of the main pancreatic duct. The cancer invasion was confined to a relatively small area. It was difficult to definitively determine whether the lesion represented partial invasion or an intraepithelial lesion.

Clinician's comment: A cyst initially measuring 8 mm in diameter in the head of the pancreas grew to 20 mm in diameter over a period of 5 years and 6 months and was therefore resected. This was an invaluable case in which the patient with a branch-duct type intraductal papillary-mucinous tumor was followed up by periodic checkups for over 5 years. A repeat CT showed that during the 2-year period after the lesion was first detected, the cystic part of the lesion had contracted, with the appearance of a pericystic low-density area that had increased gradually in size with time ; the cyst eventually reduced in size to a 2-cm low-density area over a period of 5 years and 6 months. There was the possibility, retrospectively, that carcinomatous invasion had already begun 2 years after the discovery of the lesion in the course of the follow-up, inasmuch as histopathologic studies demonstrated that the low-density area had already become invasive carcinoma, for the most part. This was an important case suggesting the possibility that the invasive carcinoma had rather started to grow with contraction of the cyst, whereas contraction of the cystic part of a lesion found during the course of follow-up did not represent contraction of the lesion.

Case 7 Main-duct type intraductal papillary-mucinous adenoma (IPMA) showing typical morphologic features

Case : A man in his 70s
Chief complaint : Asymptomatic (serum amylase elevation)
Family history : Hepatic cancer in his younger brother and gastric cancer in his younger sister
Past history : Pulmonary tuberculosis at age 27 and known diabetic since age 55, receiving oral medication
Smoking and drinking history : Drinking, moderate daily consumption of alcohol ; smoking (−)
Present illness : In August 1987, he was noted to show an increased serum level of amylase at a nearby hospital where he was being followed up for the treatment of diabetes mellitus ; an abdominal computed tomography (CT) revealed a mass in the body of the pancreas.
  He was admitted to our hospital for medical workup in early November.
Ultrasonography (US) of the abdomen (Fig. 1) : A cystic hypoechoic mass was revealed in the body of the pancreas, contiguous with the caudal aspect of the main pancreatic duct.
Contrast-enhanced CT of the abdomen (Fig. 2) : A cystic hypoechoic area with a nonhomogeneous internal density was noted in the body of the pancreas (closer to the head of the pancreas).
Endoscopic findings of the duodenal papilla (Fig. 3) : The orifice of the papilla of Vater was slightly open longitudinally.
Endoscopic retrograde cholangiopancreatography (ERCP) findings (Fig. 4) : The main pancreatic duct showed cystiform dilatation, with an internal radiolucency in the body of the pancreas (closer to the head of the pancreas).
Surgical procedure (Fig. 5) : Distal pancreatectomy was performed in mid-January 1988 (operation time, 3 hours 40 minutes ; blood loss, 450 g).
Findings on laparotomy (Fig. 6) : A grayish-white area with reddening was seen in the anterior aspect of the body of the pancreas.
Findings in the anterior aspect of the resected specimen (Fig. 7) : The body of the pancreas close to the stump of the pancreas was somewhat swollen, but there was no exposure of the tumor.
Finding of the mucus in the main pancreatic duct at the stump of the pancreas (Fig. 8) : Viscous mucus was retained in the main pancreatic duct.
Pancreatoscopic findings of the resected specimen (Fig. 9) : Agminate milky-white salmon roe-like microelevations, with superficial reddening, were seen on the main pancreatic duct epithelium.
Pancreatographic findings of the resected specimen (Fig. 10) : There was cystiform dilatation, with irregular margins, of the main pancreatic duct in the body of the pancreas in the vicinity of the stump of the pancreas. Presence of mural nodules was suspected.
Postoperative course : The patient survived for 2 years 2 months after the surgery.

Blood Cell Counts	
WBC	5,800 /μL
RBC	4.05×10^6 /L
Hb	13.0 g/dL
Ht	38.8 %
Plt	211×10^3 /μL

Tumor Markers	
CEA	3.8 ng/mL
CA19-9	43.6 U/mL
Elastase 1	293 ng/dL

Biochemistry	
TP	7.1 g/dL
T-Bil	0.4 mg/dL
ALP	171 U/L
GOT	16 U/L
GPT	18 U/L
Amy	255 U/L
Glu	111 mg/dL
BUN	18 mg/dL
Crea	0.54 mg/dL

I. Imaging Findings

Fig. 1 US of the abdomen

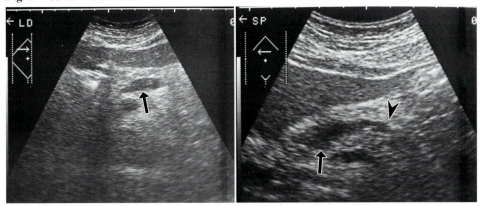

A 3-cm cystic hypoechoic mass was observed in the body of the pancreas (→), showing continuity to the caudal aspect of the main pancreatic duct (➤).

Fig. 2 Contrast-enhanced CT

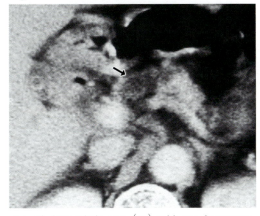

A cystic hypoechoic area (→) with non-homogeneous internal density was noted in the body of the pancreas (localized rather close to the head of the pancreas).

Fig. 3 Endoscopy of the duodenal papilla

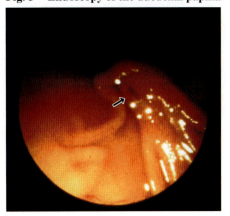

The orifice of the papilla of Vater was slightly open longitudinally (→).

Fig. 4 ERCP

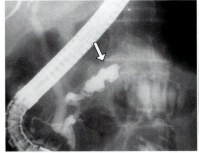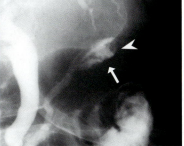

The main pancreatic duct was cystically dilated (→), with an internal radiolucency (➤), in the body of the pancreas (closer to the head of the pancreas).

II. Surgical Findings

Fig. 5 Surgical findings

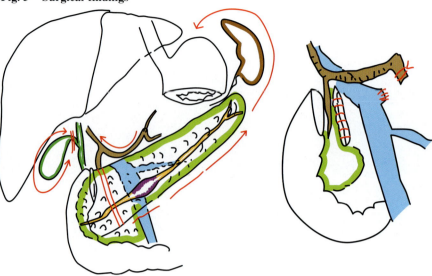

Fig. 6 Laparotomy findings

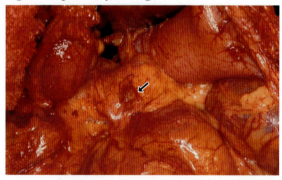

A grayish-white area (→) with reddening was seen on the anterior aspect of the body of the pancreas.

This lesion felt solid during the operation, so that the possibility of invasive carcinoma was considered. From the correlation with the histologic findings, however, it was thought to correspond to the circumscribed pancreatitic lesion in the vicinity of the tumor.

Fig. 7 Resected specimen (anterior aspect)

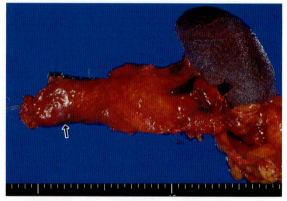

The body of the pancreas close to the stump of the pancreas was mildly swollen (→), but there was no exposure of the tumor.

Fig. 8 Mucus secreted from the main pancreatic duct at the stump of the pancreas

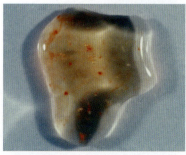

Viscous mucus accumulated in the main pancreatic duct

Fig. 9 Pancreatoscopy of the resected specimen

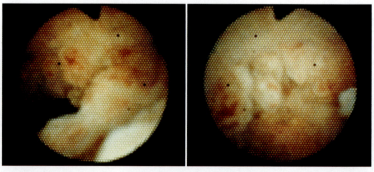

Agminate milky-white salmon roe-like microelevations, with superficial reddening, were noted on the epithelium of the main pancreatic duct.

Case 7 Main-duct type intraductal papillary-mucinous adenoma (IPMA) showing typical morphologic features

Fig. 10 Pancreatography of the resected specimen

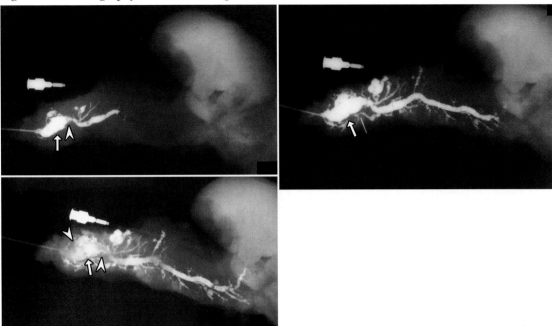

Cystiform dilatation (→) of the main pancreatic duct was observed in the body of the pancreas, close to the stump of the pancreas, and the dilated duct had irregular margins, which led us to suspect the presence of mural nodules (➤).

III. Pathological Findings

Fig. 11 Pathologic dissection diagram of the resected specimen

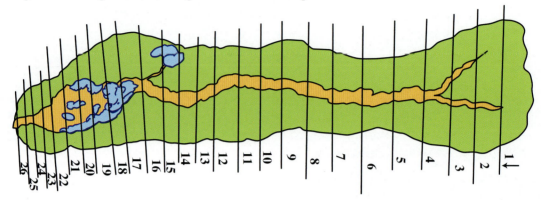

Blue part : papillary adenoma

Fig. 12 Findings of the cut surfaces of the resected specimen

1. Photograph of the cut surfaces of all sections of the resected specimen

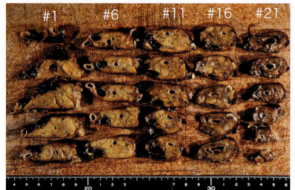

2. Photograph of the cut surfaces of sections #16 to 22

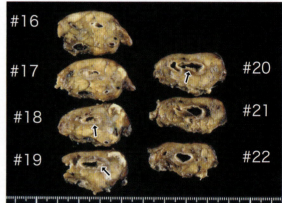

An intraductal papillary elevation (→) was noted in the distended main pancreatic duct.

3. Photograph of the cut surface of section #17

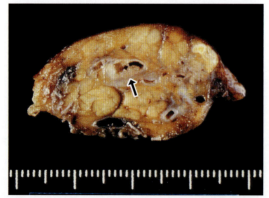

An intraductal papillary elevation (→) was noted in the main pancreatic duct.

4. Photograph of the cut surface of section #18

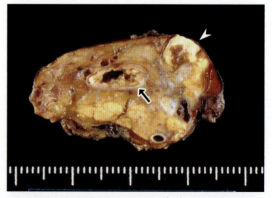

An intraductal papillary elevation (→) was noted in the main pancreatic duct with a circumscribed yellowish-white pancreatitic lesion (➤) in its vicinity.

Case 7 Main-duct type intraductal papillary-mucinous adenoma (IPMA) showing typical morphologic features 77

Fig. 13 Findings of the cut surfaces of all sections of the resected specimen

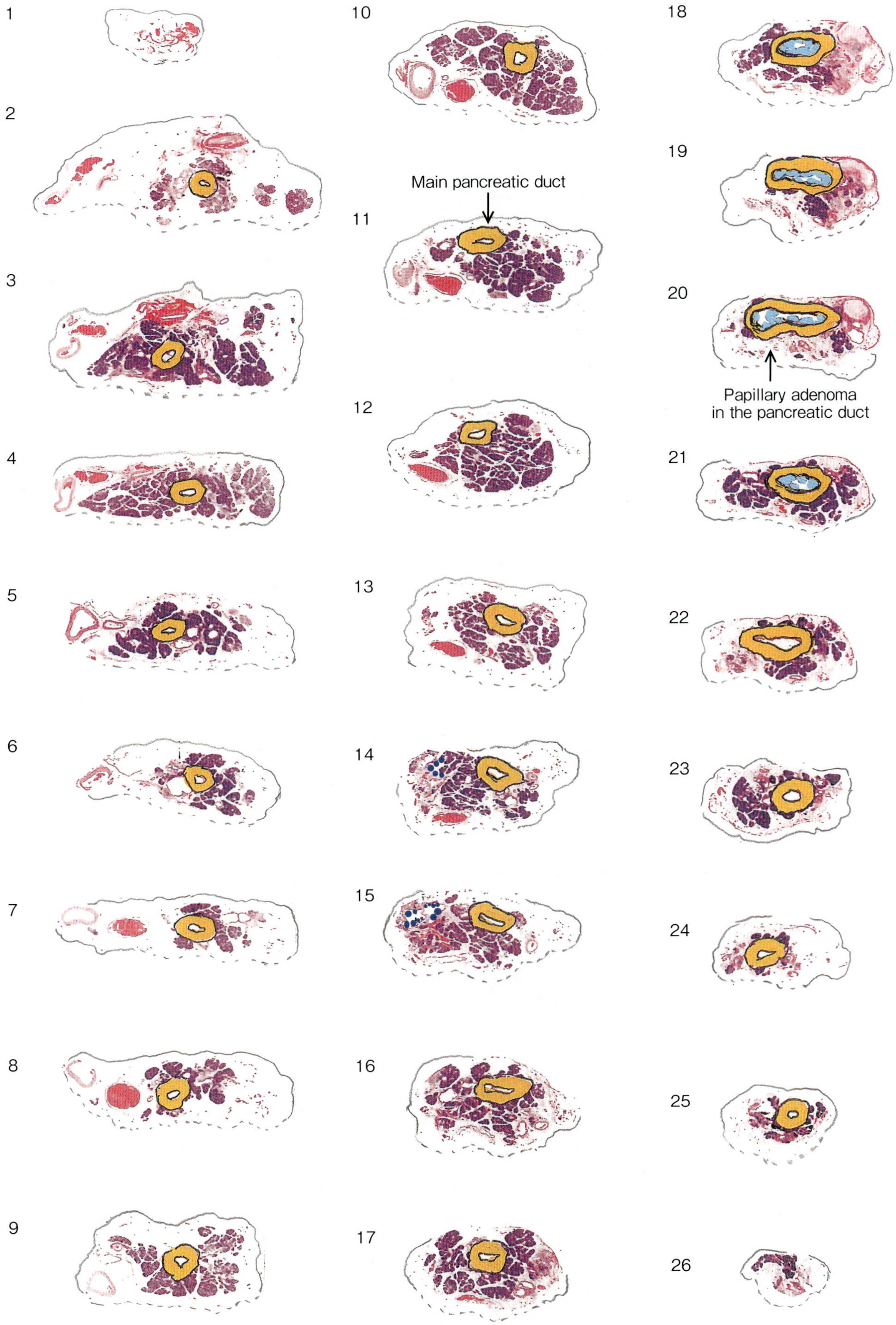

Main pancreatic duct

Papillary adenoma in the pancreatic duct

Fig. 14 Collation of the pre- and postoperative endoscopic retrograde pancreatography (ERP) images with the resected specimen

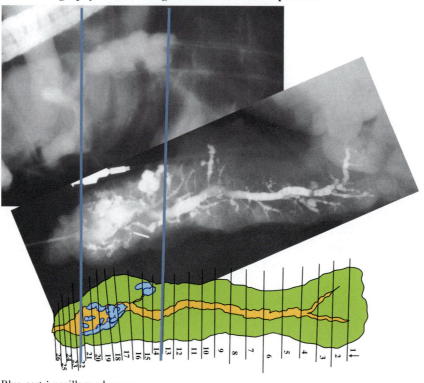

Blue part : papillary adenoma
Correlated by matching the head and tail sides of the dilated pancreatic duct
Changes were seen in the body of the pancreas and were recognized as dilatation of the main pancreatic duct and cystiform dilatation of a pancreatic duct branch. Dilatation of a branch of the pancreatic duct was also noted caudally at a site somewhat distant from the main lesion.

#16

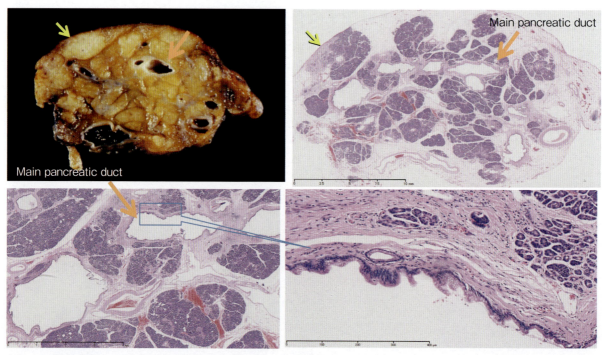

A low papillary lesion consisting of slightly atypical cells was noted in the dilated pancreatic duct branch, however, no evidence of malignancy was seen.
The yellowish-white area was a pancreatitic lesion (yellow arrow).

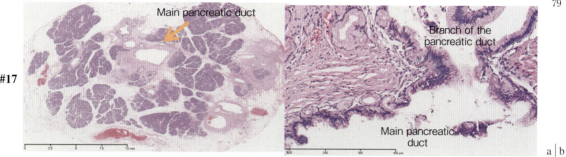

a, b. The walls of the dilated main pancreatic duct and pancreatic duct branch were composed of cells possessing abundant mucus in the cytoplasm. Cellular atypia and structural atypia were modest.

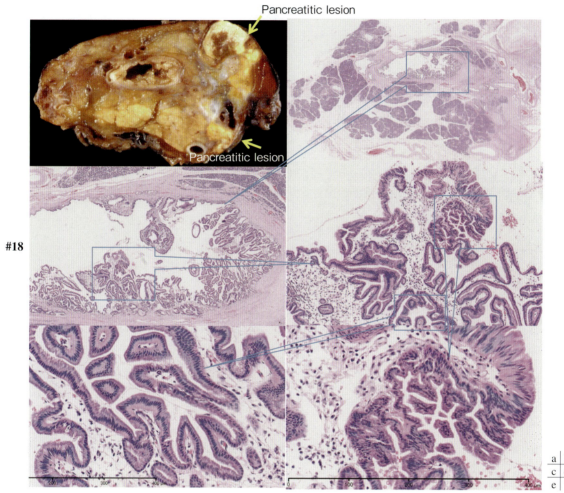

a, b, c. Papillary proliferative lesions protruding into the ductal lumen were seen in the wall of the main pancreatic duct. d, e, f. The papillary proliferative lesions showed, for the most part, slight to moderate atypia (e), however, a very limited area showed severe atypia (f) ; this region was diagnosed as a highly atypical adenoma lesion.

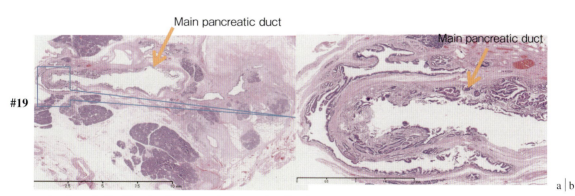

a, b. A markedly dilated main pancreatic duct, and a dilated pancreatic duct branch that appeared as if encircling the main pancreatic duct. In the walls of the dilated main pancreatic duct and dilated pancreatic duct branch, progression of a short adenoma showing papillary proliferation was noted.

Collation of the pre- and postoperative ERP images with the resected specimen

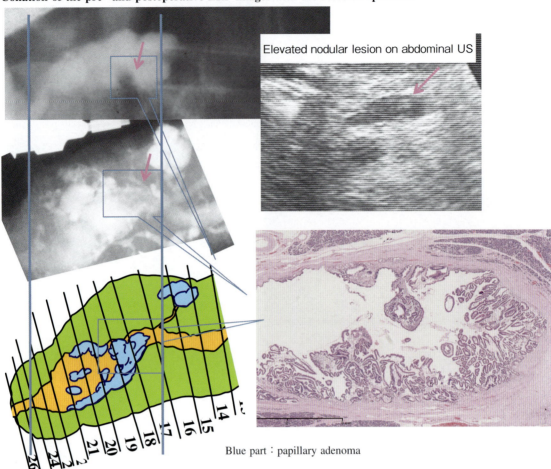

Elevated nodular lesion on abdominal US

Blue part : papillary adenoma

The low-density area or defect in the main pancreatic duct on ERP imaging coincided with the elevated nodular lesion demonstrated histopathologically. There was also the possibility that the lesion was the elevated nodular lesion observed on the abdominal US.

Histopathologic diagnosis

Intraductal papillary-mucinous neoplasm, adenoma with severe atypia, of the body of the pancreas
MPD type, 8×22 mm, N0 (0/20)

Pathologist's comment : Lesions were observed primarily in the dilated main pancreatic duct and extended slightly to involve the wall of a branch of the pancreatic duct. The lesions were moderately atypical for the most part, while adenoma with severe atypia was very rarely encountered.

Clinician's comment : This was the only benign (adenoma) case among the 12 cases of main-duct type intraductal papillary-mucinous neoplasm treated by resection at our hospital. The tumor, which was a relatively tall elevated lesion in the main pancreatic duct as viewed by gross examination of the cut surfaces of the resected specimen, was considered macroscopically as a carcinoma, but was histologically diagnosed as a papillary adenoma on account of the mild degree of atypia. At laparotomy, a grayish-white induration was felt in the front of the body of the pancreas, exactly at the site of the tumor mass ; therefore, cancerous invasion of the pancreatic capsule was considered. However, histopathologic findings negated the presence of invasive carcinoma, and the lesion was found to correspond to a circumscribed pancreatitic lesion in the vicinity of the tumor ; occlusion of a pancreatic duct branch by the intraductal tumor was considered as the cause.

Case 8 Typical intraductal papillary-mucinous adenoma (IPMA), with severe atypia, of the head of the pancreas, in which an intraductal lesion was noted in the main pancreatic duct on examination of the resected specimen by fiberoptic endoscopy

Case: A man in his 50s
Chief complaint: Asymptomatic (lesion discovered by ultrasonography [US])
Family history: No history of cancer
Past history: Not remarkable
Smoking and drinking history: Drinking, drank 180 mL of alcohol a day for 35 years ; smoking, smoked 8 cigarettes a day for 25 years
Present illness: The patient was first noted to have abnormal densities on a plain abdominal x-ray at a mass screening conducted in late September 1989.

In late November of the same year, an upper gastrointestinal endoscopic examination carried out at the Department of Internal Medicine of our hospital revealed a IIc lesion (biopsy : tub1) in the posterior wall of the cardia.

In mid-December 1989, he was admitted to our internal medicine service for endoscopic mucosal resection (EMR). Abdominal US performed prior to this procedure revealed dilatation of the main pancreatic duct ; EMR was performed, followed by a detailed checkup of the pancreas.
Abdominal US (Fig. 1) : A 6-cm cystic lesion with non-homogeneous internal echoes was noted in the head of the pancreas.
Abdominal computed tomography (CT) (Fig. 2) : A low-density mass, appearing as if internally partitioned, was visualized in the head of the pancreas.
Endoscopic findings of the duodenal papilla (Fig. 3) : The orifice of the papilla of Vater was enlarged in the transverse direction.
Findings of endoscopic retrograde cholangiopancreatography (ERCP) (Fig. 4) : Radiolucency was noted in the pancreatic duct which was dilated, with uneven thickening of the wall.
Surgical procedure (Fig. 5) : In early February 1990, pancreaticoduodenectomy was performed (operation time, 7 hours 25 minutes ; blood loss, 1,050 g).
Gross findings of the resected specimen (Fig. 6) : No tumor exposure was noted on the anterior aspect of the head of the pancreas.
Pancreatographic findings of the resected specimen (Fig. 7) : There was a filling defect and radiolucency in the dilated main pancreatic duct.
Endoscopic findings of the pancreatic duct in the resected specimen (Fig. 8) : Viscous mucus was retained in the dilated main pancreatic duct and a broad-based elevated lesion was seen.
Postoperative course: The patient survived for 18 years 4 months after the surgery.

Blood Cell Counts	
WBC	7,700 /µL
RBC	4.54×10^6 /µL
Hb	13.9 g/dL
Ht	40.5 %
Plt	278×10^3 /µL

Tumor Markers	
CEA	1.5 ng/mL
CA19-9	5.1 U/mL
Elastase 1	980 ng/dL

Biochemistry	
TP	7.1 g/dL
T-Bil	0.3 mg/dL
γ-GTP	29 U/L
ALP	253 U/L
GOT	13 U/L
GPT	34 U/L
T-chol	189 mg/dL
Amy	142 U/L
Glu	122 mg/dL
BUN	14 mg/dL
Crea	1.0 mg/dL

I. Imaging Findings

Fig. 1 Abdominal US (transverse scan)   Abdominal US (longitudinal scan)

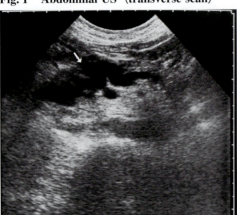
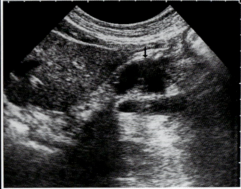

A 6-cm cystic lesion with uneven internal echoes (→) was noted in the head of the pancreas.

A cystic lesion with non-homogeneous internal echoes (→) was noted in the head of the pancreas.

Fig. 2 Contrast-enhanced CT

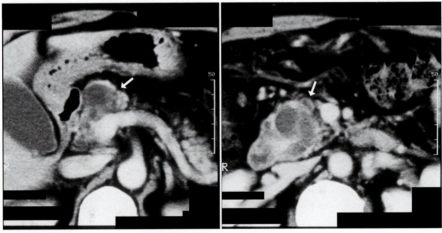

There was a low-density mass (→) appearing to have several internal partitions in the head of the pancreas.

Fig. 3 Endoscopic features of the duodenal papilla

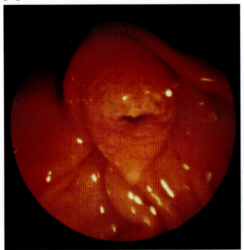

The orifice of the papilla of Vater was widened in a transverse direction.

Fig. 4 ERCP

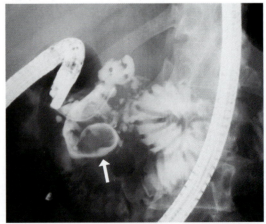

Sporadic radiolucencies were seen in the pancreatic duct which was dilated, with uneven thickening of the wall (→).

II. Surgical Findings

Fig. 5 Surgical findings

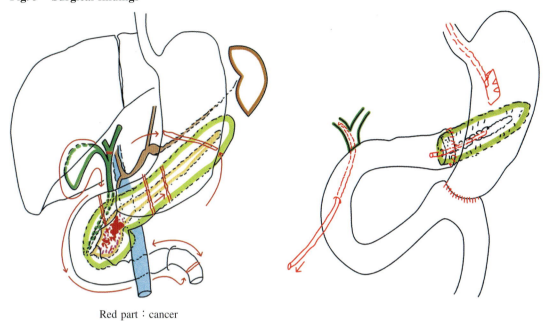

Red part : cancer

Fig. 6 Resected specimen (anterior view)

Mucus retained in the pancreatic duct of the resected specimen

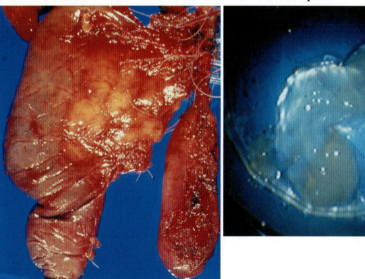

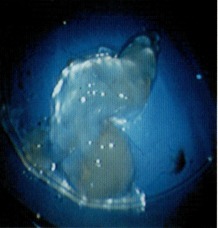

No tumor exposure on the anterior aspect of the head of the pancreas

Fig. 7　Pancreatography of the resected specimen

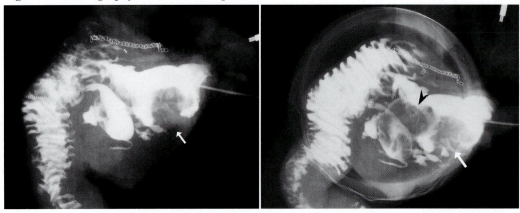

Examination of the main pancreatic duct after injection of contrast into the stump of the pancreas revealed a filling defect (→) and radiolucency (➤) in the dilated main pancreatic duct.

Fig. 8　Fiberoptic endoscopic examination of the resected pancreatic specimen

Viscous mucus (→) was present in the dilated main pancreatic duct and a broad-based elevated lesion (➤) was seen. With indigo-carmine spray, villous microprojections on the super ficial layer of the lesion became distinct.

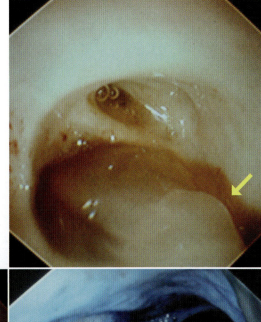

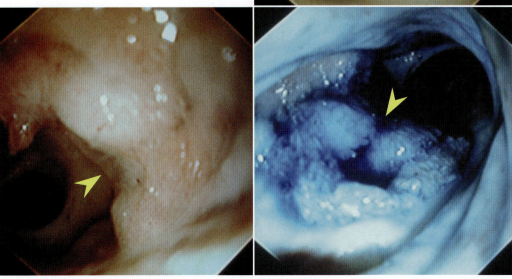

III. Pathological Findings

Fig. 9 Tissue architecture of the resected specimen

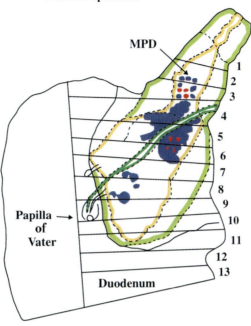

Red part : severe atypia
Blue part : slight to moderate atypia

Fig. 10 Findings of the cut surfaces of the resected specimen

1. Findings of the cut surfaces of all the sections of the resected specimen
2. Findings of the cut surfaces of sections #4 to 6

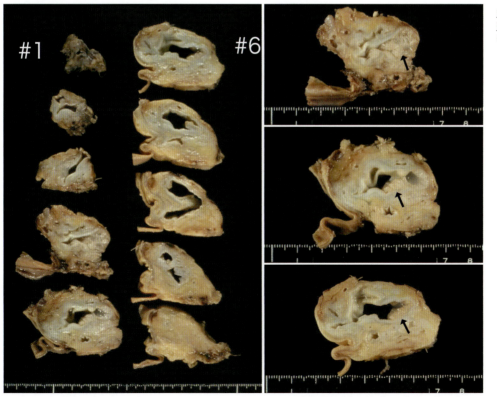

A broad-based elevated lesion (→) was noted in the distended pancreatic duct.

Fig. 11 Findings of the cut surfaces of all the sections of the resected specimen

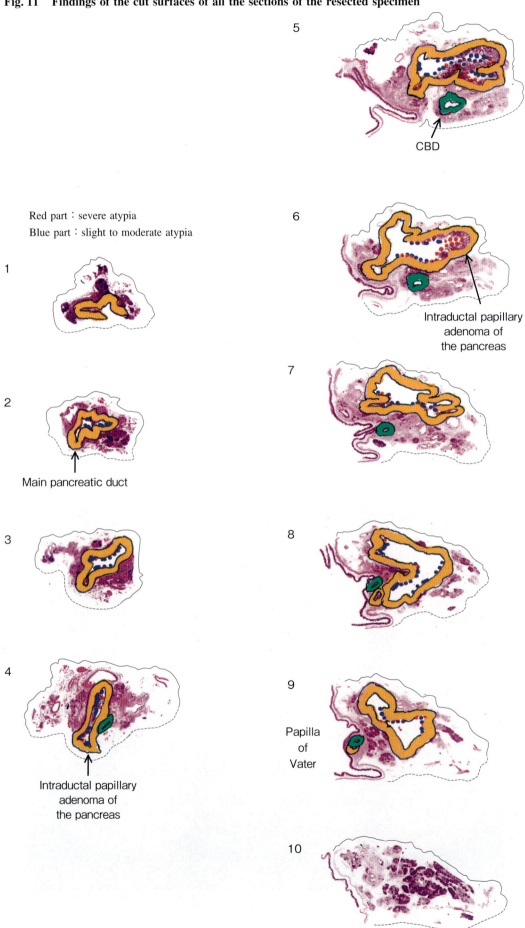

Fig. 12 Collation of the pre- and postoperative endoscopic retrograde pancreatography (ERP) images with projection views of the resected specimen

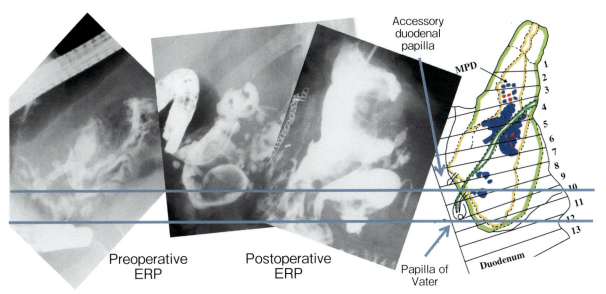

Correlated by matching the papilla of Vater and the accessory papilla
The main pancreatic duct and accessory pancreatic duct were markedly dilated and the lumen of the pancreatic duct was filled with a papillary proliferative lesion.
Red dots indicate tumors with severe atypia, and the blue dots indicate adenomas with slight to moderate atypia.
Red part : severe atypia, Blue part : slight to moderate atypia

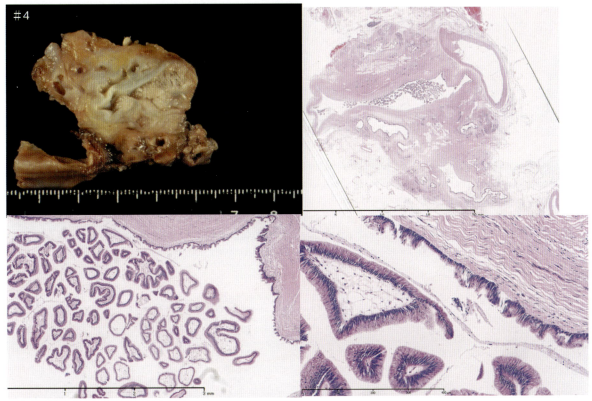

a. A papillary proliferative lesion almost totally occupying the lumen of the main pancreatic duct was noted. The papillary proliferative lesion noticeably resembled the villous structure of the large intestine. Although it was difficult to differentiate between carcinoma and adenoma in terms of the histodiagnostic degree of atypia in this case, severely atypical adenoma was diagnosed in view of the somewhat modest disturbance of polarity and relatively uniform spindle-shaped nuclei.

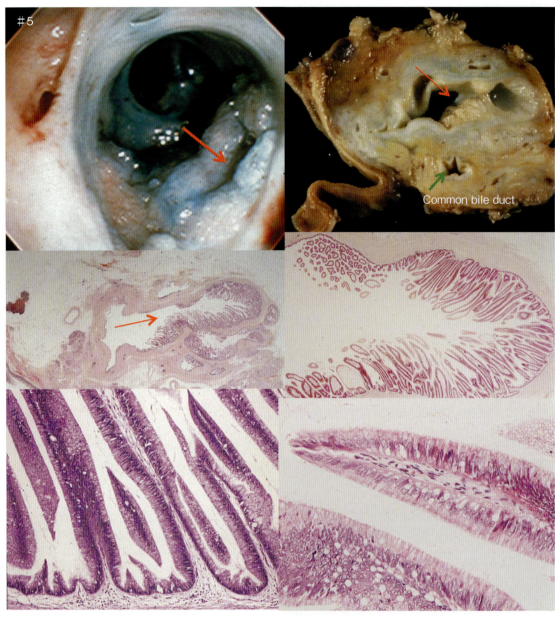

The dilated pancreatic duct was observed with a fiberoptic endoscope inserted into the stump of the main pancreatic duct in the resected specimen. The red arrow points to the site of bifurcation of the main pancreatic duct. A papillary proliferative lesion was seen extending from the main pancreatic duct to a branch of the pancreatic duct. The papillary proliferative lesion noticeably resembled the villous structure of the large intestine. Although it was difficult to differentiate between carcinoma and adenoma in terms of the histodiagnostic degree of atypia in this case, severely atypical adenoma was diagnosed in view of the somewhat modest disturbance of polarity and relatively uniform spindle-shaped nuclei.

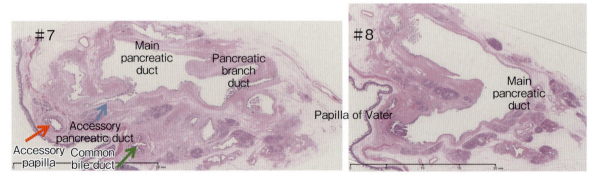

The main pancreatic duct and accessory pancreatic duct were markedly dilated and no papillary proliferative lesion was noted in the main pancreatic duct or inside the papilla of Vater.

Collation of the preoperative CT images with the histologic features

A high-density area seen in the dilated pancreatic duct on preoperative CT, reflecting the papillary proliferative lesion

Histopathologic diagnosis

Intraductal papillary-mucinous neoplasm, adenoma with severe atypia, of the head of the pancreas
Mixed type, 17×35×50 mm, N0 (0/21)

Pathologist's comment: This was a case with a pancreatic intraductal papillary proliferative lesion resembling a villous adenoma of the large intestine. Endoscopic examination of the postoperative resected specimen revealed an elevated lesion with a relatively smooth surface, which was found histopathologically to be a densely growing villous proliferative lesion. However, it was difficult on histopathological examination to definitively diagnose the tumor as a carcinoma or adenoma.

Clinician's comment: This was a case with a mixed-type pancreatic intraductal papillary-mucinous neoplasm extending from the main pancreatic duct to a branch duct in the head of the pancreas. Fiberoptic endoscopic exploration of the pancreatic duct lumen in the resected specimen, after clearing off the viscous mucus, clearly revealed a papillary tumor in the main pancreatic duct. With indigo staining, embossed microvillus elevations were seen on the tumor surface.

Case 9　A large moderately atypical intraductal papillary-mucinous adenoma (IPMA) measuring 5 cm in maximum diameter with a mural nodule

Case: A man in his 60s
Chief complaint: Asymptomatic (lesion discovered by computed tomography [CT], with patient under periodic checkup for 8 years since)
Family history: No history of cancer
Past history: Not remarkable
Smoking and drinking history: Drinking, drank a can of beer and 5 glasses of whiskey and water every day ; smoking, smoked 40 cigarettes a day for 40 years
Present illness: In March 1993, the patient underwent abdominal ultrasonography (US) at his workplace as part of a mass screening program, and was advised to undergo further workup for the upper abdomen. Thereafter, a CT of the abdomen performed at a nearby hospital revealed dilatation of the pancreatic duct. However, the patient failed to seek further medical advice at that time.
　In September 1994, the patient sought medical advice at a certain university hospital, where he was advised to undergo surgery for a Group 3 lesion detected by pancreatic duct biopsy carried out during endoscopic retrograde cholangiopancreatography (ERCP) ; however, the patient was reluctant to undergo the surgery. In late October 1994, he was admitted to our hospital for further workup. Imaging diagnostic exploration revealed a 3-cm cystic lesion in the head of the pancreas with dilatation of the main pancreatic duct.
　A Group 2 lesion was found by pancreatic duct biopsy carried out during ERCP. The patient was followed up by diagnostic imaging once or twice a year thereafter.
　In late November 1999, endosonographic examination revealed an intraductal papillary tumor, 6 mm in diameter, in Wirsung's canal.
　In late November 2000, endosonographic examination showed that the tumor diameter had increased to 10 mm.
　In mid-March 2001, pancreatoscopy and pancreatic intraductal tissue biopsy revealed a Group 3 lesion (papillary adenoma with moderate atypia). As the tumor tended to continue to grow, surgical intervention was recommended.
Abdominal US over time (Fig. 1): During the 5-year period from May 1996 to June 2001, multiple cystic lesions observed in the head of the pancreas increased gradually in size and eventually coalesced to become a large lesion.
Endosonographic examination over time (Fig. 2): Over a 7-year follow-up period, the multiloculated cystic lesion in the head of the pancreas increased in size, and a 1-cm mural nodule developed in the main pancreatic duct.
Abdominal CT over time (Fig. 3): The multiloculated cystic lesion in the head of the pancreas gradually increased in size, with progressive dilatation of the main pancreatic duct.
Magnetic resonance cholangiopancreatography (MRCP) (Fig. 4): A multiloculated cystic lesion, 4 cm in its minor axis, was noted in the head of the pancreas, with conspicuous dilatation of the main pancreatic duct in the head of the pancreas.
Endoscopic findings of the duodenal papilla (Fig. 5): The orifices of both the papilla of Vater and the accessory papillae were clearly visualized, and viscous mucus discharge was seen from the major papilla.
Pancreatoscopic findings (Fig. 6): A papillary tumor about 10 mm in diameter was noted in the dilated Wirsung's canal.
ERCP findings (Fig. 7): The main pancreatic duct was found to show cystiform dilatation and radiolucency proximal to the branching off of the accessory pancreatic duct, while the cystic lesions were only partially visualized.
Surgical procedure (Fig. 8): Pylorus-preserving pancreaticoduodenectomy was performed in early July 2001 (operation time, 12 hours 40 minutes ; blood loss, 1,010 g).
Findings in the anterior aspect of resected specimen (Fig. 9): There was no tumor exposure on the anterior aspect of the head of the pancreas.
Pancreatographic findings of the resected specimen (Fig. 10): Examination after injection of contrast into the stump of the main pancreatic duct revealed a dilated main pancreatic duct and a dilated branch of the duct with radiolucency, and then the entire coalesced multicystic lesion.
Postoperative course: The patient survived for 11 years 1 month after the surgery.

Blood Cell Counts	
WBC	5,200 /μL
RBC	4.65×10⁶ /μL
Hb	15.2 g/dL
Ht	44.8 %
Plt	271×10³ /μL

Tumor Markers	
CEA	4.7 ng/mL
CA19-9	3.0 U/mL
DUPAN-2	<25 U/mL
Elastase 1	280 ng/dL

Biochemistry	
TP	7.5 g/dL
T-Bil	0.8 mg/dL
γ-GTP	25 U/L
ALP	239 U/L
GOT	16 U/L
GPT	17 U/L
T-Chol	187 mg/dL
P-Amy	91 U/L
Glu	112 mg/dL
BUN	14 mg/dL
Crea	0.68 mg/dL

I. Imaging Findings

Fig. 1 Abdominal US over time

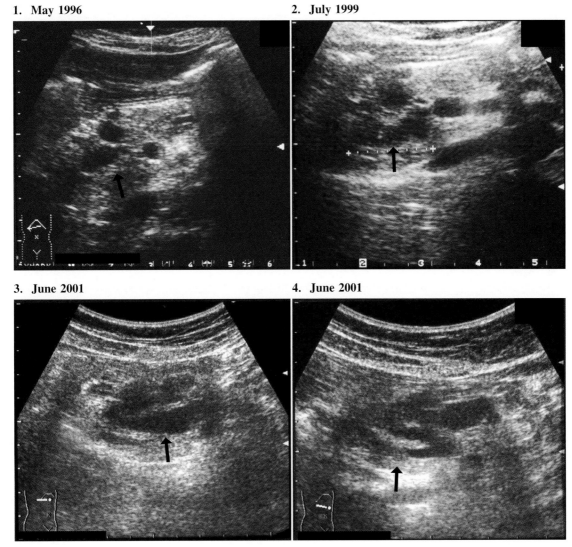

1. May 1996
2. July 1999
3. June 2001
4. June 2001

Multiple cysts in the head of the pancreas that increased gradually in size and eventually coalesced to become a large cystic lesion (→)

Fig. 2 Endosonographic examination over time
November 1994   March 2001   March 2001

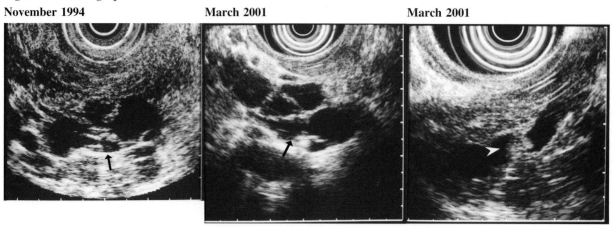

Over the 7-year follow-up period, the multiloculated cystic lesion (→) in the head of the pancreas increased in size, and a 1-cm mural nodule (►) developed in the main pancreatic duct.

Fig. 3 Abdominal CT over time
May 1996   July 1999   June 2001

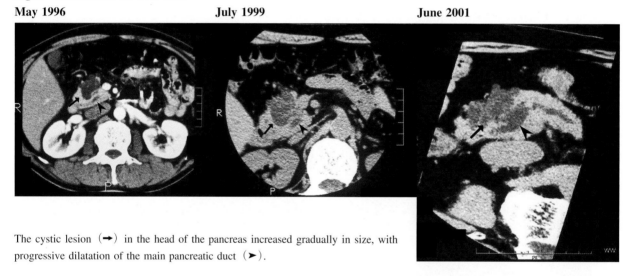

The cystic lesion (→) in the head of the pancreas increased gradually in size, with progressive dilatation of the main pancreatic duct (►).

Fig. 4 MRCP

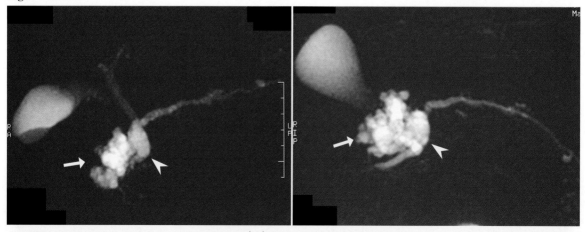

A multiloculated cystic lesion, 4 cm in its major axis (→), was noted in the head of the pancreas, with conspicuous dilatation of the main pancreatic duct (►) in the head of the pancreas.

Fig. 5 Endoscopy of the duodenal papilla

Papilla of Vater   Accessory papilla

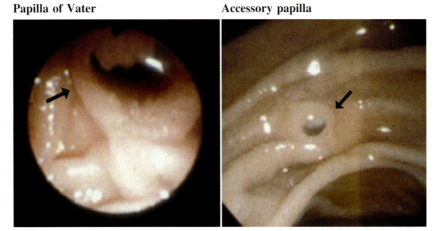

The orifices of both the papilla of Vater and the accessory papillae were clearly visualized (→), and viscous mucus discharge was seen from the major papilla.

Fig. 6 Pancreatoscopy (March 2001)

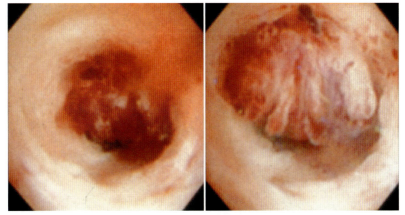

A papillary tumor 10 mm in diameter was noted in the dilated Wirsung's canal. Histopathologic examination of a biopsy specimen revealed a Group 3 lesion (papillary adenoma).

Fig. 7 ERCP

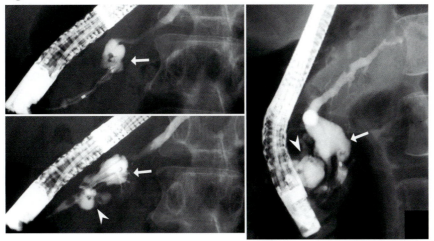

The main pancreatic duct proximal to its branching showed cystiform dilatation and a radiolucency (→). The branch (accessory pancreatic duct?) showed marked cystiform dilatation (➤), while the entire cystic lesion was not visualized.

II. Surgical Findings

Fig. 8　Surgical findings

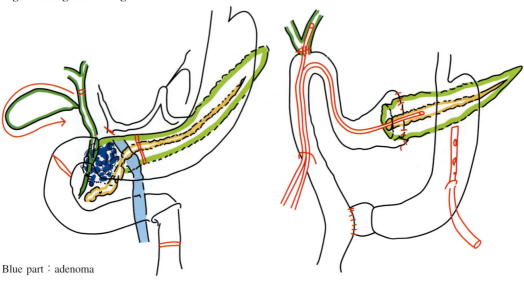

Blue part : adenoma

Fig. 9　Resected specimen (anterior aspect)

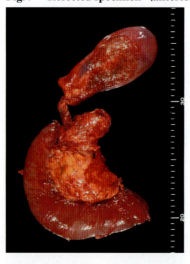

There was no tumor exposure on the anterior aspect of the head of the pancreas.

Fig. 10　Pancreatography of the resected specimen

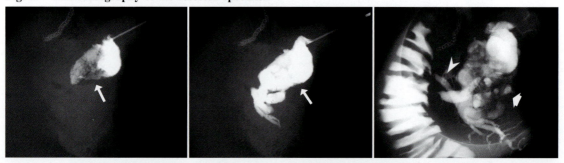

Examination after injection of contrast into the stump of the main pancreatic duct revealed a dilated main pancreatic duct with intraductal radiolucency, a dilated pancreatic duct branch (→), and then the whole coalesced multicystic lesion (⇨) and accessory pancreatic duct (➤).

III. Pathological Findings

Fig. 11 Pathologic dissection diagram of the resected specimen

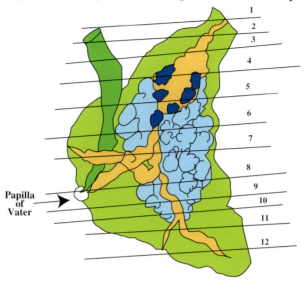

Deep blue : severe atypia, Light blue : slight to moderate atypia

Fig. 12 Findings of the cut surfaces of the resected specimen

1. Photograph of the cut surfaces of all sections of the resected specimen

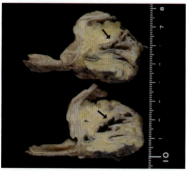

2. Photograph of the cut surfaces of sections #4 and 5

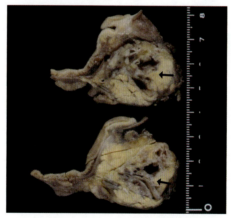

A tumor appearing as an aggregate of dilated pancreatic ducts (→), primarily situated on the ventral side of the head of the pancreas was noted.

3. Photograph of the cut surfaces of sections #6 and 7

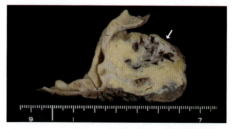

A tumor appearing as an aggregate of dilated pancreatic ducts (→) was noted.

4. Photograph of the cut surface of section #8

A tumor consisting of dilated pancreatic ducts and an aggregate of small cysts (→) was noted on the ventral side of the head of the pancreas.

Fig. 13 Findings of all the cut surfaces of the resected specimen

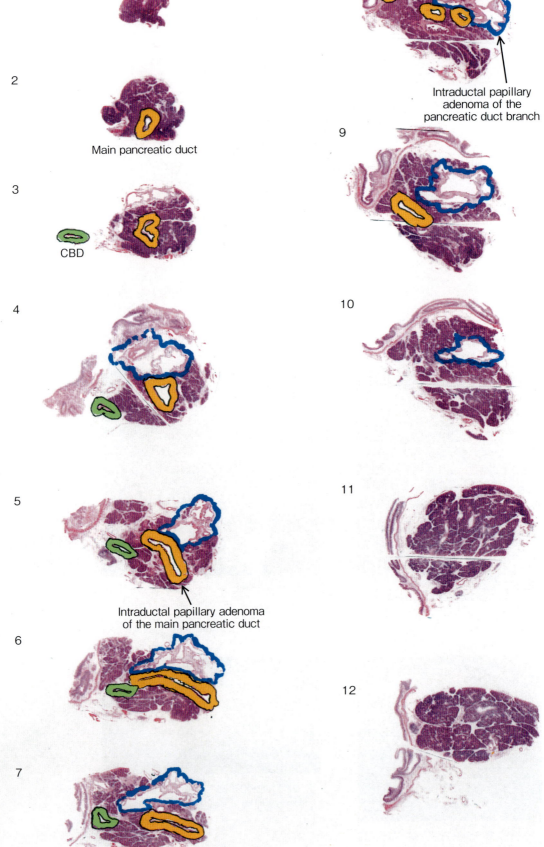

Case 9 A large moderately atypical intraductal papillary-mucinous adenoma (IPMA) measuring 5 cm in maximum diameter with a mural nodule

Fig. 14 Collation of the pre- and postoperative pancreatographs with projection views of the resected specimen

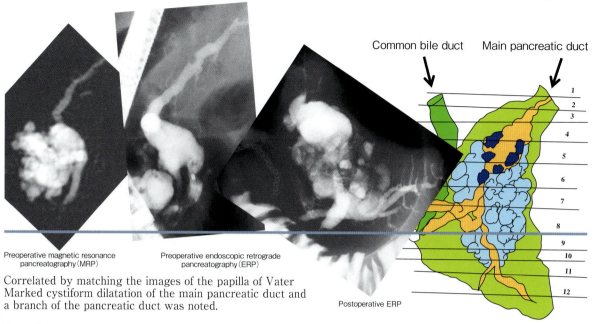

Preoperative magnetic resonance pancreatography (MRP)

Preoperative endoscopic retrograde pancreatography (ERP)

Postoperative ERP

Correlated by matching the images of the papilla of Vater
Marked cystiform dilatation of the main pancreatic duct and a branch of the pancreatic duct was noted.

Deep blue : severe atypia, Light blue : slight to moderate atypia

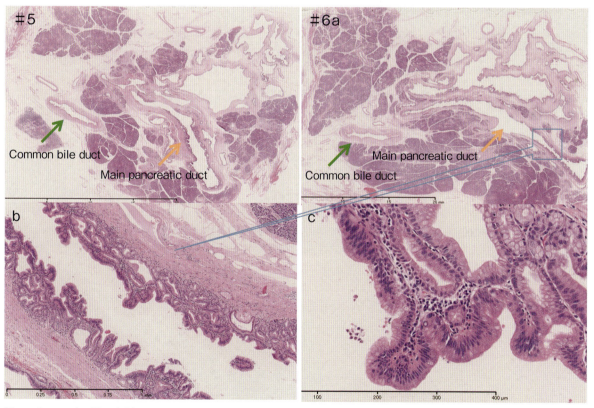

Photomicrographs #5 and #6
A markedly dilated main pancreatic duct and pancreatic duct branch were noted. An intramural small elevated lesion was seen in the main pancreatic duct. c. The elevated lesion showed a weakly atypical papillary structure.

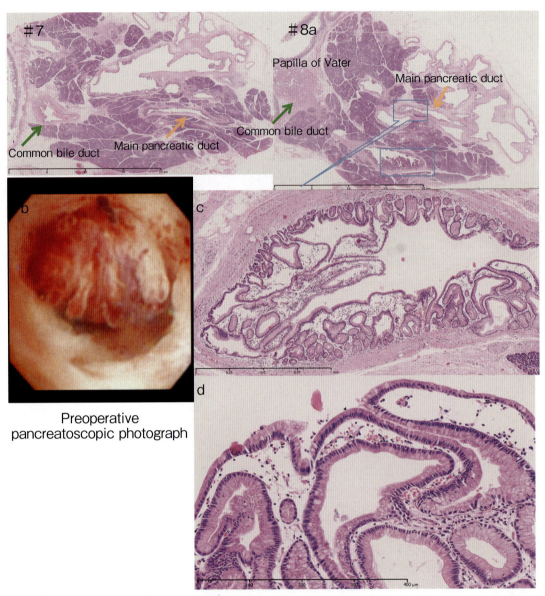

A papillary tumor measuring 10 mm in diameter observed in the dilated Wirsung's canal was considered to correspond to the region indicated by the square in #8, as viewed from its location relative to the papilla of Vater and the main pancreatic duct. The lesion was a slightly atypical papillary adenoma consisting of mucus-rich cells with cellular atypia.

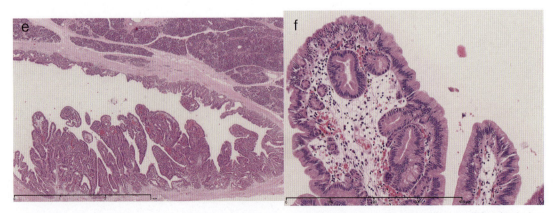

e, f. Higher magnifications of the region indicated by the square in #8a. The relatively tall papillary proliferative lesion in the dilated pancreatic duct branch was noted. The lesion was diagnosed as an adenoma with moderate atypia.

Collation of the preoperative CT image with the photomicrograph

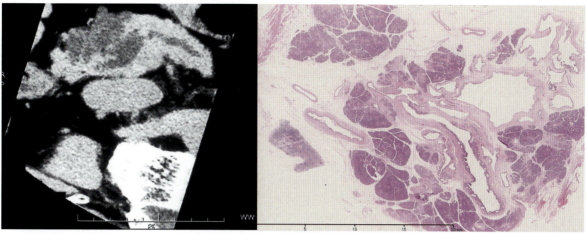

Shown here is a photomicrograph of an area proximal to the region shown in the CT image. The CT image showed cystiform dilation of the main pancreatic duct and a pancreatic duct branch. From the CT image, this region was diagnosed as a mural nodule-free flat pancreatic wall.

Histopathologic diagnosis

Intraductal papillary-mucinous neoplasm (IPMN), adenoma with moderate atypia, of the head of the pancreas
Mixed type, 50×30×25 mm, N0 (0/9)

Pathologist's comment: This was a typical IPMN associated with pancreatic duct dilatation. A relatively short elevated lesion was noted extensively in the dilated wall of the pancreatic duct. For the most part, the atypia was mild. However, a tall elevated lesion with moderate atypia was observed in one part of the lesion.

Clinician's comment: This was a valuable case that had been followed up for over 8 years since the patient was first detected by US, in a mass screening program, to have dilatation of the main pancreatic duct and multilocular cysts. During the 8-year follow-up period, the dilatation of the main pancreatic duct progressed and the multilocular cyst grew gradually in size. Although the patient was rather reluctant to undergo surgery, pancreatoscopic exploration revealed a 1-cm polypoid lesion in the lumen of the main pancreatic duct along with enlargement of the multilocular cysts to a coalescent cyst measuring >4 cm in diameter, and the lesion was finally resected. The tumor measured 50 mm in maximum diameter in the resected specimen. Clinically, the possibility of cancer was considered.

Case 10 Non-invasive intraductal papillary-mucinous carcinoma (IPMC) spreading across the entire pancreas

Case: A woman in her 70s
Chief complaint: Back pain
Family history: Gastric cancer in father
Past history: Surgery for appendicitis at age 26, Hashimoto's disease since age 49
Smoking and drinking history: Drinking (−); smoking (−)
Present illness: In mid-December 1987, the patient developed back pain (predominantly on the right side) and was admitted to a local facility. Abdominal ultrasonography (US) revealed abnormalities of the pancreas. The first visit of the patient to our hospital was in early March, 1988.
In late March, the patient was admitted to our hospital for detailed examination.
Hypotonic duodenography (Fig. 1): Evidence of extramural compression from outside the wall was noted on the medial side of the duodenal C loop.
Abdominal computed tomography (CT) (Fig. 2): Cystic dilatation of the pancreatic duct was visible from the head to the body of the pancreas.
Angiography (Fig. 3): Dorsal pancreatic arteriography revealed signs of compression and extension at the periphery of the arteries in the pancreatic head and body regions.
Endoscopic findings of the duodenal papilla (Fig. 4): The major and minor papillae were swollen, with the opening enlarged and showing mucus discharge.
Findings on endoscopic retrograde cholangiopancreatography (ERCP) (Fig. 5): The main pancreatic duct was dilated, with irregularities of the lumen. Probably because of the mucus in the pancreatic duct, the pancreatic tail was not completely filled with the contrast material.
Surgical procedure (Fig. 6): In early May, pancreatoduodenectomy (subtotal) was carried out (operation time, 5 hours 45 minutes; blood loss, 1,007 g).
Macroscopic observation of the resected specimen (Fig. 7): Swollen major and minor papillae were visible on the mucosal plane of the duodenum.
Findings on main pancreatic duct (pancreatic head) endoscopy of the resected specimen (Fig. 8): Papillary elevated lesions were visible almost along the full circumference of the main pancreatic duct lumen.
Findings on stereoscopic microscopy of the main pancreatic duct epithelium in the resected specimen (Fig. 9): Minimal salmon roe-shaped elevations were seen at a high density on the main pancreatic duct epithelium.
Findings on pancreatography of the resected specimen (Fig. 10): The main pancreatic duct was diffusely dilated, with irregularity of the lumen and shadow defects.
Postoperative course: The patient died of debility 3 years and 3 months after the surgery.

Blood Cell Counts	
WBC	11,600 /μL
RBC	3.58×10^6 /μL
Hb	11.2 g/dL
Ht	33.6 %
Plt	169×10^3 /μL

Tumor Markers	
CEA	5.8 ng/mL
CA19-9	7.5 U/mL
Elastase 1	124 ng/dL

Biochemistry	
TP	5.5 g/dL
Alb	2.8 g/dL
T-Bil	0.5 mg/dL
γ-GTP	13 U/L
ALP	278 U/L
GOT	15 U/L
GPT	14 U/L
T-chol	206 mg/dL
Amy	751 U/L
Glu	102 mg/dL
BUN	11 mg/dL
Crea	0.56 mg/dL

I. Imaging Findings

Fig. 1 Hypotonic duodenography

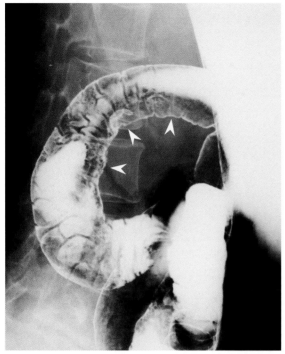

Evidence of extramural compression from outside the wall was noted on the medial side of the duodenal C loop (▶).

Fig. 3 Angiography

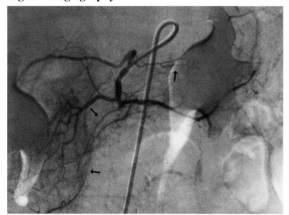

Dorsal pancreatic arteriography showed signs of compression and extension at the periphery of the arteries in the pancreatic head/body region (→).

Fig. 2 Contrast-enhanced CT

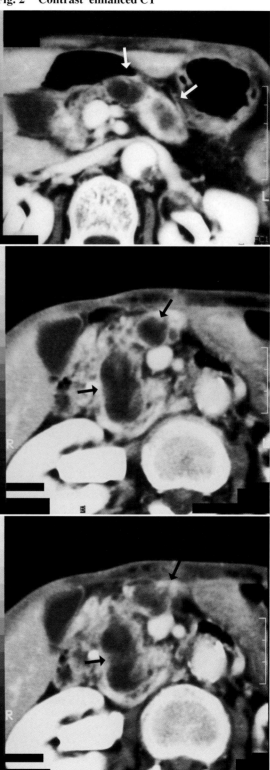

Cystic dilatation of the pancreatic duct was visible from the head to the body of the pancreas (→).

Fig. 4 Endoscopic findings of the duodenal papilla

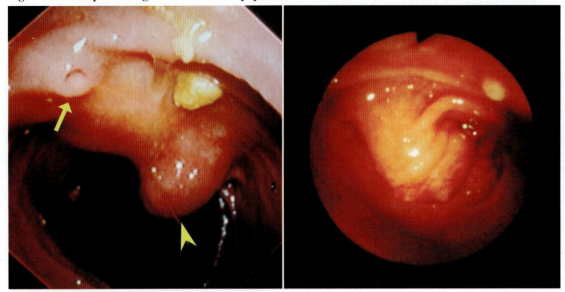

The minor papilla and major papilla (▶) were swollen, with enlargement of the opening (→).

Swollen major papilla

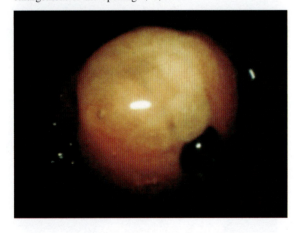

Viscous mucus discharge was seen from the major papilla.

Fig. 5 ERCP

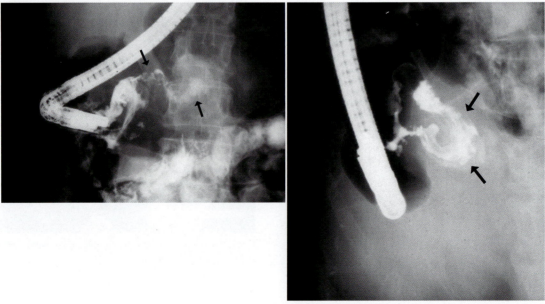

Dilatation and irregularity of the lumen (→) of the main pancreatic duct were seen. Probably because of the mucus in the pancreatic duct, the contrast material did not fill the pancreatic duct in the body/tail region completely.

II. Surgical Findings

Fig. 6 Surgical findings

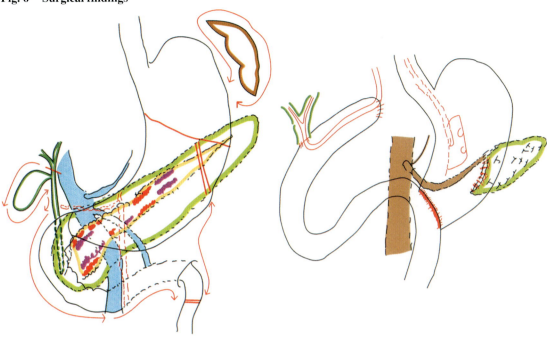

Fig. 7 Photographs of the resected specimen (after duodenotomy)

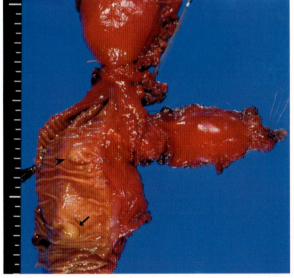

On the mucosal surface of the duodenum, the swollen major papilla (→) and minor papilla (➤) were visible.

Close-up image of the duodenal mucosal plane

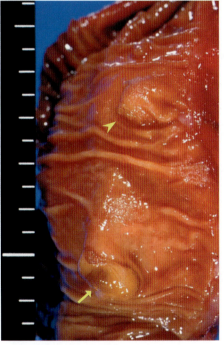

Both the major papilla (→) and the minor papilla (➤) were swollen, and the openings were enlarged. Mucus was found to be adhering to the opening of the major papilla.

Fig. 8 Main pancreatic duct (pancreatic head) endoscopy of the resected specimen

Fig. 9 Stereoscopic endoscopy of the main pancreatic duct epithelium of the resected specimen

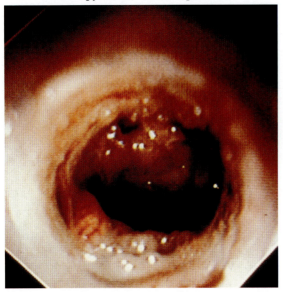

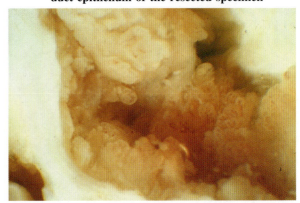

Minimal salmon roe-shaped elevations were densely distributed on the main pancreatic duct epithelium.

Approximately full-circumferential papillary elevated lesions were visible inside the main pancreatic duct.

Fig. 10 Pancreatography of the resected specimen

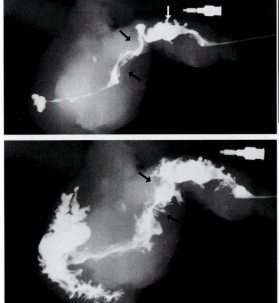

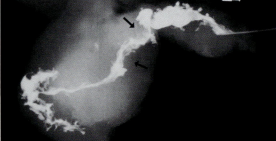

Following injection of the contrast material into the stump of the main pancreatic duct in the pancreatic tail, a diffusely dilated main pancreatic duct with irregular luminal width and shadow defects (→) was visualized.

III. Pathological Findings

Fig. 11 Tissue architecture of the resected specimen

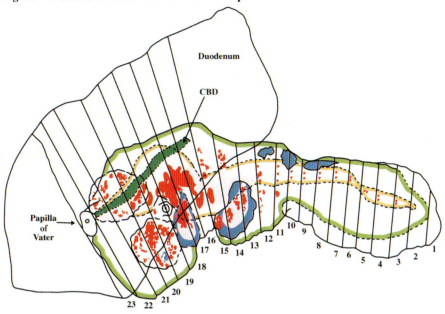

Red part : cancer, Blue part : adenoma

Fig. 12 Findings of the cut surfaces of the resected specimen
1. Photograph of the cut surfaces of all the sections of the resected specimen

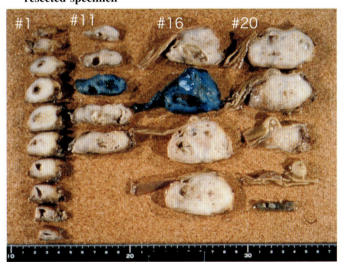

Fig. 12 Findings of the cut surfaces of the resected specimen

2. Findings of the cut surface of section #13

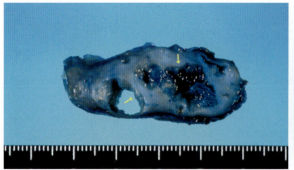

A papillary tumor and blob of mucus were visible in the dilated main pancreatic duct and pancreatic duct branches (→).

3. Findings of the cut surface of section #14

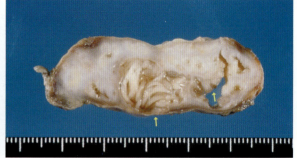

Papillary tumors were visible in the dilated main pancreatic duct and pancreatic duct branches (→).

4. Findings of the cut surface of section #17

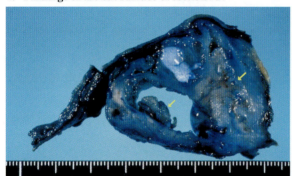

Papillary tumors were visible in the dilated main pancreatic duct and pancreatic duct branches (→).

5. Findings of the cut surface of section #20

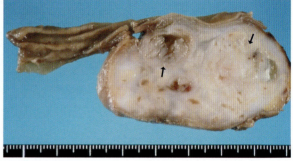

Papillary tumors were visible in the dilated main pancreatic duct and pancreatic duct branches (→).

Fig. 13 Findings of the cut surfaces of all the sections of the resected specimen

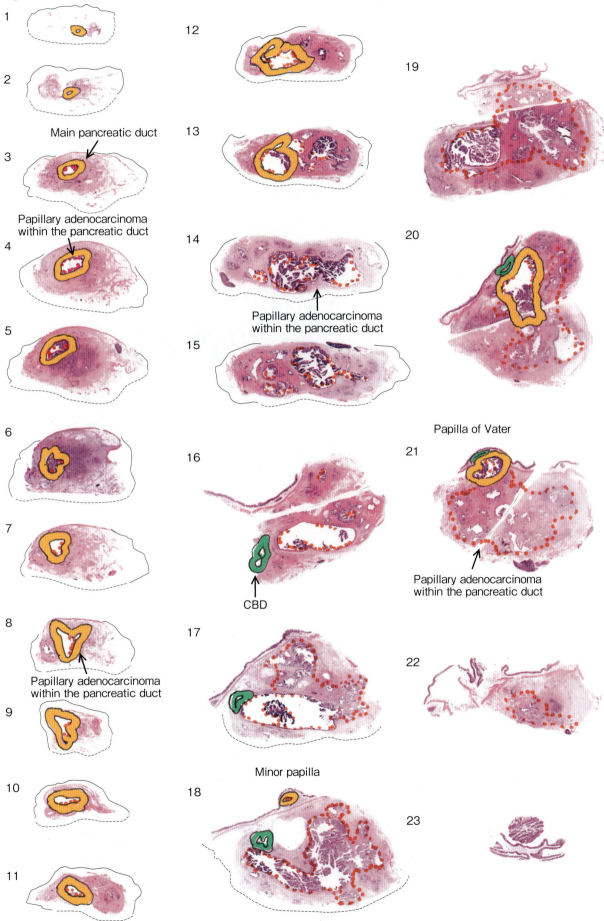

Fig. 14 Collation of the pre- and postoperative endoscopic retrograde pancreatography (ERP) images with projection views of the resected specimen

The major lesions were located in the main pancreatic duct and pancreatic duct branches from the head to the body of the pancreas. The pancreatic duct was markedly dilated and filled with papillary proliferative lesions, making one-to-one matching of the images and histological findings difficult. Matching was done in the following way : Area A, dilated segment of the main pancreatic duct at the tail ; Area B, stenosed segment of the main pancreatic duct in the tail ; Area C, dilated segment of the main pancreatic duct in the body ; Area D, stenosed segment of the main pancreatic duct in the head.

Area A : Dilated segment of the main pancreatic duct in the tail region of section #3

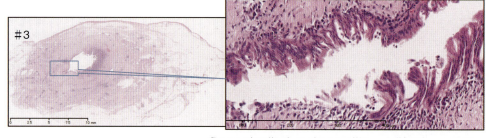

Cancer visualized as short papillary proliferation spreading within the main pancreatic duct

Area B : Stenosed segment of the main pancreatic duct in the tail region of section #6

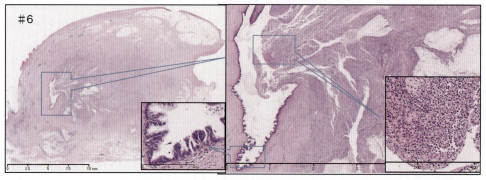

The main pancreatic duct was narrowed by inflammatory granulation tissue. The epithelium remaining in the wall of main pancreatic duct lumen showed cancerous short papillary proliferation.

Area C : Dilated segment of the main pancreatic duct in the pancreatic body of section #11 to 15

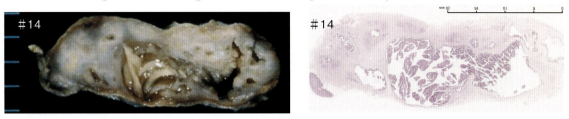

The main pancreatic duct and pancreatic duct branches were markedly dilated, with tall papillary proliferation visible in the pancreatic duct lumen at the pancreatic head, which was cancerous.

Area D : Minor papilla in the pancreatic head in section #18

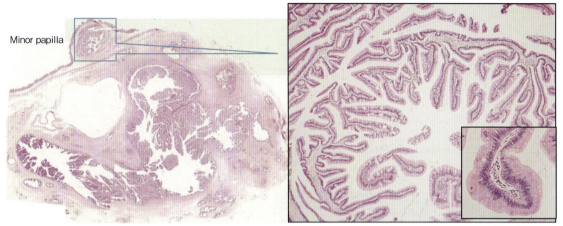

The main pancreatic duct, accessory pancreatic duct and pancreatic duct branches were markedly dilated, each filled with papillary proliferative lesions. The papillary proliferative lesions had spread to the accessory pancreatic duct. b. The papillary proliferative lesion within the accessory pancreatic duct was an adenoma.

Area D : Major papilla in the pancreatic head in section #21

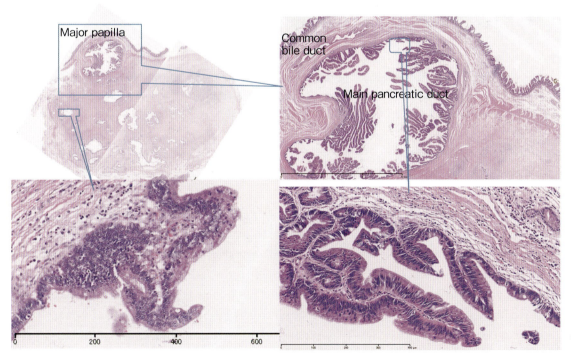

The main pancreatic duct and the pancreatic duct branches were dilated, each filled with papillary proliferative lesions. The papillary lesions had spread to the major papilla (#21a). The epithelium of the pancreatic duct branches showed cancer (c) and adenoma lesions, while the papillary proliferative lesions within the major papilla were highly atypical adenoma lesions (d).

Collation of the preoperative images with the histologic features

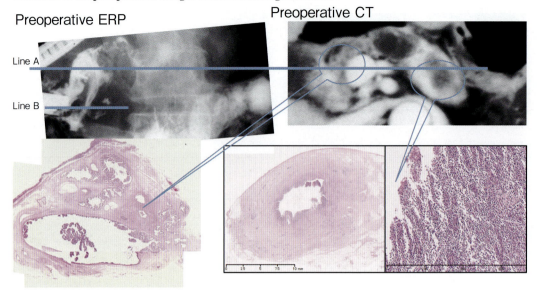

The high-density area on the CT images of the pancreatic head corresponded to the papillary proliferative lesions. The high-density area around the dilated pancreatic duct in the pancreatic body/tail corresponded to the granulation tissue accompanied by marked inflammatory cell infiltration.

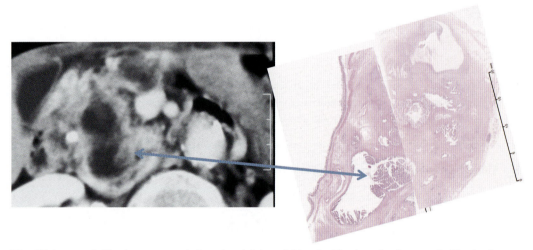

The CT image of this site corresponded to the vicinity of Line B. The low-density area inside the lumen corresponded to the dilated pancreatic duct, and the slightly high density area corresponded to the papillary proliferative lesions.

Histopathologic diagnosis

Intraductal papillary-mucinous neoplasm (IPMN), carcinoma with adenoma, non-invasive, of the whole pancreas
Mixed type, 70×40×35 mm, N0 (0/38)

Pathologist's comment : Papillary proliferative lesions, spreading almost throughout the entire pancreas, were visible. Strongly atypical lesions were predominant, and adenomatous lesions were sporadically seen. The residual pancreatic parenchyma was almost atrophic. This is a typical case of IPMN spreading across the entire pancreas.

Clinician's comment : Diagnostic imaging revealed extensive dilatation of the main pancreatic duct and pancreatic duct branches from the head to the body of the pancreas. Because of marked mucus production, both the major and minor duodenal papillae were swollen, with their openings enlarged and discharged viscous mucus, thus showing the typical features of an intraductal papillary tumor. Subtotal pancreatectomy of the cranial side was carried out, leaving only 5 cm of the pancreatic tail (the part not showing main pancreatic duct dilatation) unresected. The stump was closed and joined to the stomach by suturing.